VIROLOGY RESEARCH PROGRESS

AVIAN INFLUENZA

MOLECULAR EVOLUTION, OUTBREAKS AND PREVENTION/CONTROL

Virology Research Progress

Additional books in this series can be found on Nova's website under the Series tab.

Additional e-books in this series can be found on Nova's website under the e-book tab.

Allergies and Infectious Diseases

Additional books in this series can be found on Nova's website under the Series tab.

Additional e-books in this series can be found on Nova's website under the e-book tab.

VIROLOGY RESEARCH PROGRESS

AVIAN INFLUENZA

MOLECULAR EVOLUTION, OUTBREAKS AND PREVENTION/CONTROL

KYLE M. TAYLOR
AND
BRUCE O'CONNOR
EDITORS

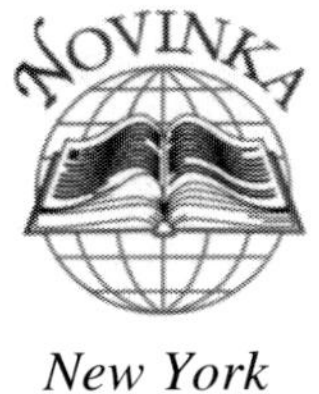

New York

For permission to use material from this book please contact us:
Telephone 631-231-7269; Fax 631-231-8175
Web Site: http://www.novapublishers.com

NOTICE TO THE READER

Additional color graphics may be available in the e-book version of this book.

Library of Congress Cataloging-in-Publication Data

ISBN: 978-1-62417-415-5

Library of Congress Control Number: 2012954581

Published by Nova Science Publishers, Inc. † New York

CONTENTS

PREFACE

Avian influenza or bird flu refers to "influenza caused by viruses adapted to birds." Of the greatest concern is the highly pathogenic avian influenza (HPAI). Most human contractions of the avian flu are a result of either handling dead infected birds or from contact with infected fluids. In this book, the authors discuss the molecular evolution, outbreaks and prevention/control of avian influenza. Topics include the risk assessment of highly pathogenic avian influenza virus infections through water; biosecurity measures against highly pathogenic avian influenza (HPAI) in free-range flocks and commercial poultry in developing countries; outbreak control and viral evolution of the highly pathogenic H5N1 avian influenza in Thailand; and the changes in perceptions and attitudes that were identified in a follow-up survey conducted when bird flu was not the focus on widespread media coverage in Australia.

Chapter 1 – Wild waterfowl are considered as the natural reservoir of all influenza A virus subtypes, including H5N1. Influenza A viruses replicate preferentially in the gastrointestinal tract of waterfowl, high concentrations are excreted in feces, and the viruses can be transmitted via the fecal-oral route among the waterfowl. Infected waterfowl can contaminate open water bodies, including drinking water sources and recreational areas, and the oral ingestion or aspiration of water containing influenza A virus could be a possible mode of transmission to humans. Quantitative microbial risk assessment (QMRA) framework is a powerful tool to understand how to control pandemics mediated by environmental reservoirs or human-to-human transmission (e.g. calculating risk of infection due to a low dose). Essential steps in the QMRA process are, exposure assessment and dose-response analysis. Recently, H5N1 influenza risk assessment models (1) to estimate the probability of human infection from H5N1 through water and (2) to describe mortality of experimental animals exposed to H5N1 (time-dependent dose-response model) were developed. These models will be useful to evaluate the risks of infection under various transmission scenarios and contribute to prevention of a future human influenza pandemic caused by this lethal virus.

Chapter 2 – The emerging and re-emerging of infectious diseases over the last few decades demonstrate the potential for introduction of epidemic illnesses such as avian influenza through global migration of animals and humans. Recent outbreaks of a highly pathogenic avian influenza (HPAI) strain H5N1 in Asia and Africa have caused severe impacts on the poultry industries worldwide, both through bird mortality and morbidity and the resultant trade restrictions and negative demand shocks. There is also a considerable global concern that the virus could mutate into a form that can be passed between humans, which poses a significant risk of leading to a global pandemic. The risk 'mitigation' measures and risk 'propagation' practices in free-range flocks could influence introduction and maintenance of low pathogenic avian influenza (LPAI) with consequent depression in immunity of the free-range flocks, mutation and development of HPAI. These enormous potential liabilities have led to significant global investments in the disease prevention and control. However, poultry producers have roles to play in the prevention and control of avian influenza.

In this study, a review biosecurity measures practice in free-range flocks and commercial poultry operations in developing countries. The scientific literature on the prevention/control of highly pathogenic avian influenza of the past years is reviewed. The review findings are plausible as birds from free-range flocks have more opportunities of contact with wild birds that serve as reservoirs of low-pathogenic avian influenza strains than the commercial poultry, thus providing them with constant challenge of flock immunity. The development of efficient and effective biosecurity measures against avian influenza on commercial farms requires adequate placements of barriers to provide segregation, cleaning and disinfection, while concerted community established sanitary measures are needed for free-range poultry flocks in the developing economies. Good biosecurity levels on the farms and in the flocks ultimately lower costs in the production cycle, and flock welfare is always enhanced.

Chapter 3 – Thailand is known for its success in controlling the highly pathogenic H5N1 avian influenza epidemic. Despite the explosive outbreak in 2003-2004 similar to other countries in the East and Southeast Asian region, the epidemic was bought down under control in 2006 with the elimination of infectious sources by "stamping out", strengthened biosecurity measures, and periodic active surveillance as the main control strategies. The initial epidemic in 2003-2005 involved mainly medium to large scale farming, resulting in massive economic loss. After 2006, sporadic cases occurred seasonally in backyard poultry in certain repeated outbreak areas involving limited number of poultry. The last animal outbreak was reported in 2008, and the last indigenous human case was detected in 2006. The reduction of viral population size was also evidenced by the reduced viral sequence diversity after 2006. The viral sequences showed little changes without evidences of positive selection during this low level endemic period and no known human-adapted mutations were observed. Similarity of viral sequences among outbreak seasons indicated that the virus was maintained in a local reservoir between outbreak seasons. Virus of similar lineage was occasionally isolated from local wild birds and migratory birds. Although some of these birds migrate in a route covering Southeast Asia to the epidemic hot spots in Central Asia, the similarity of viral sequences in these birds to the local virus suggested that the birds acquired the virus locally rather than carrying new viruses into the country. The small reservoir size in a limited area suggested that the virus can be eradicated from the country. While the current situation in the country is well under control, new kindle from undetected local reservoirs and import of new viral strains through human or wildlife activities are still a threat.

Chapter 4 – A survey of 200 Australian adults in May 2006 found reasonable levels of awareness, but low levels of concern, regarding bird flu. This paper reports on the changes in perceptions and attitudes that were identified in a follow-up survey conducted when bird flu was not the focus of widespread media coverage.

A computer assisted telephone survey was conducted in August and September 2006. A total of 5,565 eligible households were contacted and 805 interviews completed (response rate of 14.5%).

Bird flu fell from fourth to seventh most-frequently mentioned infectious disease. The majority of respondents were in favour of the government implementing quarantine procedures in the event of an outbreak, but less in favour of the government closing schools and offering people experimental vaccines or drugs. Respondents had low levels of awareness of preventive actions, but were generally willing to engage in these when they were identified.

We found that within four months of the initial high levels of concern bird flu was "off the radar" for the majority of the Australian population. One of the most important findings was that the general public appeared willing to engage in the appropriate preventive and protective behaviours, in the 'unlikely' event of a bird flu outbreak in Australia, but was lacking awareness of what these behaviours are.

Our results suggest that the Australian government will face a number of significant communication challenges in the event of an influenza pandemic. Not the least of these will be the need to communicate risk at the same time as educating people about appropriate preventive behaviours.

In: Avian Influenza ISBN: 978-1-62417-415-5
Editors: K. M. Taylor and B. O'Connor

Chapter 1

RISK ASSESSMENT OF HIGHLY PATHOGENIC AVIAN INFLUENZA VIRUS INFECTIONS THROUGH WATER

***Masaaki Kitajima*[1] *and Toru Watanabe*[2]**
[1]Department of Soil, Water and Environmental Science,
The University of Arizona, Tucson, Arizona, US
[2]Department of Food, Life and Environmental Sciences,
Yamagata University, Yamagata, Japan

ABSTRACT

Wild waterfowl are considered as the natural reservoir of all influenza A virus subtypes, including H5N1. Influenza A viruses replicate preferentially in the gastrointestinal tract of waterfowl, high concentrations are excreted in feces, and the viruses can be transmitted via the fecal-oral route among the waterfowl. Infected waterfowl can contaminate open water bodies, including drinking water sources and recreational areas, and the oral ingestion or aspiration of water containing influenza A virus could be a possible mode of transmission to humans. Quantitative microbial risk assessment (QMRA) framework is a powerful tool to understand how to control pandemics mediated by environmental reservoirs or human-to-human transmission (e.g. calculating risk of infection due to a low dose). Essential steps in the QMRA process are, exposure assessment and dose-response analysis. Recently, H5N1 influenza risk assessment models (1) to estimate the probability of human infection from H5N1 through water and (2) to describe mortality of experimental animals exposed to H5N1 (time-dependent dose-response model) were developed. These models will be useful to evaluate the risks of infection under various transmission scenarios and contribute to prevention of a future human influenza pandemic caused by this lethal virus.

1. INTRODUCTION

Influenza A viruses are members of the family *Orthomyxoviridae*, which comprises enveloped viruses with segmented, negative-sense RNA genomes (Wright et al. 2007). Based on the antigenicity of the two surface glycoproteins, hemagglutinin (HA) and neuraminidase (NA), influenza A viruses are currently divided into 16 HA and 9 NA subtypes, designated as H1-H16 and N1-N9. All subtypes of influenza A viruses have been isolated from waterfowl, and they are the natural reservoir of influenza A viruses and asymptomatic virus carriers (Webser et al. 1992). Avian influenza A viruses replicate not only in the respiratory tract but also in the gastrointestinal tract in waterfowl and are thus shed in high concentrations in the feces (Webster et al. 1978). Avian influenza viruses have been isolated from water bodies where waterfowl gather and can persist for a long period of time in water. Infected waterfowl can contaminate open water bodies, including drinking water sources and recreational areas, and the oral ingestion or aspiration of water containing influenza A virus could be a possible mode of transmission to humans, although most human infection cases of H5N1 highly pathogenic avian influenza virus had a history of very close contact with infected birds, and inhalation of infectious droplets or aerosols was probably the most common route of infection (Brankston et al. 2007).

This chapter discusses the potential risk of influenza virus infection through water and the prevention/control of waterborne influenza outbreaks.

2. INFLUENZA VIRUS IN WATER

Detection Methods

Virus concentration is an essential step to detect viruses at low levels in water. Roepke et al. (1989) modified the **vir**us **ad**sorption-**el**ution (VIRADEL) utilizing 1MDS filter (Cuno, Meriden, CT, USA), which was used for the detection of human enteric viruses in large volumes of water (Farrah et al. 1976), and evaluated for the concentration of influenza virus from water. The VIRADEL procedure (primary concentration) was combined with the chicken erythrocyte adsorption technique (secondary concentration), which was able to concentrate influenza virus for up to 3200-fold from 100-L tap water (Roepke et al., 1989).

However, influenza virus is not recovered as efficiently as enteric viruses, probably because the structure of influenza virus is different from that of enteric virus. The methods based on virus adsorption onto formalin-fixed chicken blood cells have been proposed for concentration of influenza viruses in environmental water (Khalenkov et al. 2008, Dovas et al. 2010), sometimes in combination with the filter adsorption (Sivanandan et al. 1991).

Several methods have been employed to detect influenza viruses in water. Isolation in embryotic specific-pathogen-free (SPF) eggs followed by reverse transcription-polymerase chain reaction (RT-PCR) assay is highly sensitive for detection of infectious virus particles (Khalenkov et al. 2008). Early techniques of isolating the influenza virus from lake water used unconcentrated water samples along with isolation in allantoic or amniotic cavities of embryonated chicken eggs or in tissue culture, such as Madin–Darby canine kidney (MDCK) cells, followed by hemagglutination inhibition or virus neutralization assays to confirm the presence of virus. Later, immunofluorescence methods and PCR-based assays were applied. At present, virus detection methods that use different PCR-based techniques, such as real-time PCR detection of different segments of influenza virus genes by using specific primers and probes with simultaneous subtyping (Stone et al. 2004), are most popular.

In our recent evaluation, H1N1 and H5N3 influenza viruses were not recovered as efficiently as enteric viruses by Mg-method (Katayama et al. 2002), Al-method (Haramoto et al. 2004), and 1-MDS method, because the structure of influenza virus is different from that of enteric virus. Modified Mg-method, which utilizes elution buffer (pH 7.9) containing 0.5% Tween 80, provided reasonably high recovery efficiency of up to 17% (Kitajima 2011).

Occurrence

Previous studies describing the occurrence of influenza viruses in water are summarized in Table 1.

Table 1. Occurrence of influenza viruses in water

Detection methods	Water type	Detection of indigenous influenza viruses				Rerefence
		Subtype	Country/Region	Titer[a]	Detection	
None	Lake water	H7N2, H4N1	Canada	NA	Egg isolation	Hinshaw et al. 1979
1MDS	Surface water	H13N2	Minnesota	NA	Egg isolation	Sivananda n et al. 1991
Chicken erythrocytes	Pond/ lake water	H4N6, H3N8, H7N3	Alaska	$10^{1.8}$ to $10^{2.8}$ EID_{50}/ml	Egg isolation	Ito et al. 1995
None	Lake ice	H1	Russia	NA	RT-nested PCR	Zhang et al. 2006
NanoCeram	Pond water	Non-H5 AIV	France	3×10^{1} to 9×10^{3} $TCID_{50}$-equivalent/L	RT-qPCR	Deboosere et al. 2011
PEG precipitation	Lake water	H10N8	China	NA	Egg isolation	Zhang et al. 2011
Ultrafiltration	Sewage	Influenza A	Netherlands	2.6×10^{5} copies/L	RT-qPCR	Heijnen and Medema 2011
None	Surface water	Influenza A	California	C_T value: 38.9±0.2	RT-qPCR	Hénaux et al. 2012

[a]EID_{50}, 50% egg infectious dose; $TCID_{50}$, 50% tissue culture infectious dose; C_T, cylcle threshold.

The concentrations of influenza viruses excreted by infected birds in environmental water are considered to be quite low because of dilution with water bodies. However, it has been reported that influenza viruses can be detected from lake water even without concentration when a number of wild waterfowls are present (Hinshaw et al. 1979, Webster et al. 1992). Influenza A viruses have been isolated from unconcentrated lake water on the shores of Canadian lakes where wild ducks had congregated before winter migration (Hinshaw et al. 1979). A recent study reported that 12 out of 597 (2.0%) unconcentrated water samples collected from 10 wetlands in two regions of the California Central Valley were positive for influenza A virus RNA by RT-qPCR targeting matrix gene (Hénaux et al. 2012).

Table 2. Detection of influenza viruses in human feces

Virus type	Remarks	References
Seasonal A	• Viral RNA was detected in feces by RT-PCR.	Wootton et al. 2006
Influenza B	• Viral RNA was detected in feces by RT-PCR.	Wootton et al. 2006
H3N2	• Viral RNA was detected in feces by real-time RT-PCR; 1.7×10^4~8.0×10^7 copies/g-stool (n=6).	Chan et al. 2009
H5N1	• Infectious virus was detected in a rectal swab. • Viral RNA was also detected by real-time RT-PCR; 9.8×10^4 copies/ml-rectal swab (n=1).	de Jong et al. 2005
H5N1	• Viral RNA in fecal swab was detected by real-time RT-PCR; 8.6×10^2~1.7×10^6 copies/ml-VTM[a] (n=4). Infectious virus was also detected in fecal swabs.	Buchy et al. 2007
H1N1 2009 pdm	• Viral RNA was detected by real-time RT-PCR; 1.44×10^4 copies/ml-stool (mean, n=4). Infectious virus was also detected in a stool. • Viral RNA was detected in urine by real-time RT-PCR but infectious virus was not detected.	To et al. 2010
H1N1 2009 pdm	• Viral RNA was detected from fecal samples by real-time RT-PCR in 16/65 (24.6%) of hospitalized individuals.	Yoo et al. 2010

[a]VTM, virus transfer medium.

However, viable influenza virus was not isolated with embryonating eggs, which suggests that the influenza virus concentration in water was low and/or the virus was inactivated by environmental factors, such as temperature and UV (Hénaux et al. 2012). The VIRADEL procedure was used to concentrate influenza virus, and low pathogenic avian influenza virus (H13N2) was isolated from 500 L of lake water in Minnesota (Sivanandan et al. 1991). Zhang et al. (2011) isolated an H10N8 influenza virus from lake water in China using polyethylene glycol (PEG) precipitation. It is possible that influenza viruses are frozen and preserved in ice or in lake water. Zhang et al. (2006) detected H1 influenza virus gene from 20 out of 373 ice meltwater samples collected from three northeastern Siberian lakes that are visited by large numbers of migratory birds. Results obtained in this study indicate that influenza A virus RNA is preserved in high concentrations in lake ice, which might facilitate genetic reassortment and/or recombination between the viruses shed during the previous year and the viruses newly acquired by birds that spent winter months in the south (Zhang et al. 2006). Since several studies reported viral shedding in stool of patients infected with influenza viruses (Table 2), influenza viruses could potentially be present in municipal sewage water via feces excreted by infected individuals. In April 2009, a novel influenza virus A (H1N1) emerged in Mexico and California. Typical flu-like symptoms as well as gastrointestinal symptoms (vomiting, diarrhea, and abdominal pain) were also frequently observed in patients infected with pandemic influenza A (H1N1) 2009 virus, and this virus was detected in feces of infected patients (Yoo et al. 2010, To et al. 2010). Heijnen and Medema (2011) reported the results of monitoring of influenza viruses in sewage and surface water; although influenza A viruses were detected, the pandemic influenza A (H1N1) virus was not detected. Similarly, raw sewage samples collected over a year in Tokyo, Japan and Arizona, US were tested for the presence of influenza virus matrix (M) gene by real-time RT-PCR, but no amplification was observed from any samples (Kitajima M, unpublished data). These results imply that the water cycle does not play a relevant in spreading influenza A virus, including the pandemic influenza A (H1N1) virus.

Persistence

Avian influenza viruses can persist for a long period of time in water, although little information is available for the subtype H5N1. In a study by Ito et al. (1995) that obtained 7 positives for influenza A virus out of 13 water samples (54%) collected at a lake where ducks were nesting in summer. The positive rate remained high (14%) in the following autumn after ducks had migrated, which suggests that the viral particles were able to persist in water.

Table 3. Persistence of influenza viruses in water

Water type	Subtype	Temperature (°C)	pH	Salinity (ppt)	Findings	Reference
River water	H3N6	22	6.8	-	Infective up to 4 days	Webster et al. 1978
River water	H3N6	0	6.8	-	Infective over 30 days	Webster et al. 1978
Distilled water	H3N8, H4N6, H6N2, H12N5, H10N7	17		0	Infective for 207 days	Stallknecht et al. 1990a

Table 3. (Continued).

Water type	Subtype	Temperature (oC)	pH	Salinity (ppt)	Findings	Reference
Distilled water	H3N8, H4N6, H6N2, H12N5, H10N7	28		0	Infective for 102 days	Stallknecht et al. 1990a
Distilled water	H6N1	17	8.2	0	Infective for 100 days	Stallknecht et al. 1990b
Distilled water	H6N1	28	8.2	20	Infective for 9 days	Stallknecht et al. 1990b
Distilled water	H5N1	17	7.4	0	16 to 26 days for 1 log reduction	Brown et al. 2007
Distilled water	H5N1	17	7.4	15	14 to 30 days for 1 log reduction	Brown et al. 2007
Distilled water	H5N1	17	7.4	30	14 to 19 days for 1 log reduction	Brown et al. 2007
Distilled water	H1N1pdm	4	6.5	0	Infective for 716 days	Dublineau et al. 2011
Distilled water	H1N1pdm	4	6.5	5	Infective for 449 days	Dublineau et al. 2011
Distilled water	H1N1pdm	4	6.5	35	Infective for 106 days	Dublineau et al. 2011
Distilled water	H1N1pdm	4	6.5	270	Infective for 34 days	Dublineau et al. 2011
Distilled water	H1N1pdm	35	6.5	0	Infective for 8 days	Dublineau et al. 2011
Distilled water	H1N1pdm	35	6.5	5	Infective for 10 days	Dublineau et al. 2011
Distilled water	H1N1pdm	35	6.5	35	Infective for 6 days	Dublineau et al. 2011
Distilled water	H1N1	4	6.5	0	Infective for 605 days	Dublineau et al. 2011
Distilled water	H1N1	4	6.5	5	Infective for 240 days	Dublineau et al. 2011
Distilled water	H1N1	4	6.5	35	Infective for 28 days	Dublineau et al. 2011
Distilled water	H1N1	4	6.5	270	Infective for 40 days	Dublineau et al. 2011
Distilled water	H1N1	35	6.5	0	Infective for 9 days	Dublineau et al. 2011
Distilled water	H1N1	35	6.5	5	Infective for 9 days	Dublineau et al. 2011
Water type	Subtype	Temperature (°C)	pH	Salinity (ppt)	Findings	Reference
Distilled water	H1N1	35	6.5	35	Infective for 3 days	Dublineau et al. 2011

Previously reported laboratory-scale influenza virus persistence experiments are summarized in Table 3. Webster et al. (1978) reported that the low-pathogenic influenza viruses remain infectious in lake water for more than 30 days at 0 °C and for up to 4 days at 22 °C. Stallknecht et al. (1990a) used five low-pathogenic avian influenza viruses (H3N8, H4N6, H6N2, H12N5, and H10N7) and showed that infectivity of virus in water was retained for up to 207 days at 17 °C and 102 days at 28 °C.

In a study by Stallknecht et al. (1990b), effects of water temperature (17 °C and 28 °C), salinity (0 ppt and 20 ppt), and pH (6.2, 7.2, 8.2) on persistence of H6N2 avian influenza virus were evaluated; estimated persistence of infectivity was longest at 17 °C, 0 ppt, pH 8.2 (100 days) and shortest at 28 °C, 20 ppt, pH 8.2 (9 days). Recent studies revealed that H5 and H7 avian influenza viruses, including highly pathogenic strains, have the ability to persist in water with wide variety of temperature and salinity for extended periods of time (Brown et al., 2007). In general, influenza viruses persist longer at low temperatures (<17 °C), fresh to brackish salinities (0 to 20,000 ppm), and slightly basic pH (7.4 to 8.2) (Brown et al. 2009).

3. Risk Assessment of Avian Influenza Infections

Quantitative Microbial Risk Assessment (QMRA)

The term "risk" is often defined as the probability that a substance or situation would produce harm under specified conditions therefore microbial risk means the probability of infection or disease for those who are exposed to water, food, air, fomites and in general outdoor and indoor environments contaminated by pathogenic microorganisms.

Quantitative Microbial Risk Assessment (QMRA) is the method for assessing such microbial risks but in a broader sense, according to QMRA Wiki led by the Center for Advancing Microbial Risk Assessment (CAMRA), it is a framework and approach that brings information and data together with mathematical models to address the spread of microbial agents through environmental exposures and to characterize the nature of the adverse outcomes.

QMRA is usually made through four steps derived from the chemical risk assessment paradigm:

(1) Hazard identification to identify the target microorganism and the endpoint of assessment (infection, illness or death).
(2) Dose-response assessment to analyze quantitative relationship between the likelihood of endpoint (i.e. response) and the level of exposure to the target microorganism (i.e. dose) on the basis of the data from human volunteer studies. This dose-response assessment is arguably the most important step in QMRA paradigm since it is sometimes impossible due to the lack of data from such human feeding studies for the target microorganism.
(3) Exposure assessment to identify affected population, to determine (or assume) the exposure pathways and environmental fate and transport of the target microorganism, to calculate the amount, frequency and length of time of exposure, and then to estimate dose, occasionally with its distribution, for the affected population.
(4) Risk characterization to estimate the magnitude of risk with its uncertainty by integrating results of dose-response assessment and exposure assessment.

The risk estimated as a conclusion of QMRA is used for risk management and risk communication which is an interactive process of exchange of information and opinion on risk among risk assessors, risk managers, stakeholders and general public.

Historically QMRA has been developed for waterborne pathogenic microorganisms, mainly aiming at establishment of water quality standards and evaluation of water treatment and disinfection system. Since the first report by Haas (1983), dose-response models for various pathogenic microorganisms were proposed by fitting either exponential or beta-Poisson model to data from human volunteer studies (Haas et al. 1999). These biologically plausible models are applicable not only to waterborne but also to airborne pathogenic microorganisms and models for *Bacillus anthracis* (Bartland et al. 2008), SARS coronavirus (Watanabe et al. 2010), seasonal influenza virus (Watanabe et al. 2012) and H5N1 influenza virus (Kitajima et al. 2011) and so on have been developed in recent years.

The goal in assessing risks is to develop and implement strategies that can monitor and control the risks (or safety) and allows one to respond to emerging diseases, outbreaks and emergencies that impact the safety of water, food, air, fomites and in general our outdoor and indoor environments, according to QMRA wiki. In case of airborne pathogenic microorganisms like influenza virus, QMRA would enable us to evaluate effects of supposed control measures (e.g., face mask and hand washing) by analyzing both a relationship between pathogen and human in dose-response assessment, and microbiological and physical phenomena important for disease transmission in exposure assessment.

Risk of Infection Through Water

Potential modes of transmission to humans of avian influenza through water include oral ingestion and inhalation of contaminated water. There is no epidemiological evidence on the incidence of human infections with avian influenza viruses through drinking water but it is theoretically possible. Quantitative risk assessments were performed in the Netherlands and Japan to estimate a risk of avian influenza virus infection through consumption of contaminated drinking water (Schijven et al. 2005, Kitajima et al. 2010). Schijven et al. (2005) estimated daily infection risks of chickens and humans due to consumption of drinking water that was contaminated with H5N1 avian influenza virus, assuming that an infected duck sheds the virus in surface water and that a portion of the shed virus passed through the drinking water treatment and reached a chicken or human. In this study, it was found that the mean daily risk of infection to an individual chicken by consumption of contaminated drinking water was low and that H5N1 infection of humans in the Netherlands from properly treated drinking water is negligible. Kitajima et al. (2010) estimated the risk of infection associated with drinking water consumption, direct contact (swimming) with contaminated surface water, and secondary-transmission via indoor air, and also demonstrated that risk of avian influenza virus infection through water, in current states, is considered to be substantially low.

The potential for exposure to avian influenza viruses is greatest in open water bodies harboring significant number of waterfowl populations. Actually, the possibility of getting the avian influenza virus infection following swimming or bathing in water with high load of virus has been suggested by epidemiological investigations in Vietnam (Vong et al. 2009) and Cambodia (de Jong et al. 2005), which implies that swimming or bathing in household ponds is a risk factor for influenza H5N1 virus infection.

Moreover, fecal shedding of influenza viruses demonstrated by the previous studies (Table 2) would result in contamination of sewage and discharge of contaminated sewage that might contaminate surface water.

Influenza Dose-Response Models

Although human infection with H5N1 highly pathogenic avian influenza virus is of a great public health concern, dose-response model for the human infection of this virus has not been reported.

This is partly because there are no data sets describing human challenge with wild-type H5N1 virus due to its high mortality.

This situation seems common to other pathogens with a high virulence such as SARS coronavirus (Watanabe et al. 2010). Previous microbial dose-response studies on several pathogens, however, have demonstrated that data from animal experiments provide reasonable estimates for human susceptibility (Haas et al. 2000; Armstrong et al. 2007; Bartrand et al. 2008). Mice have also been widely used as mammalian models to study pathogenesis of H5N1 virus; a major advantage of this model is that infection experiments can be performed with large groups of animals, because of the relatively low cost and easy-husbandary, to achieve statistical significance (Belser et al. 2009).

Katz et al. (2000a) reported that H5N1-infected mice exhibited inflammatory cell infiltration that is also observed for human fatal cases associated with H5N1 virus infection (de Jong 2008).

Ferrets are excellent model to study pathogenesis and transmissibility of influenza viruses because their clinical symptoms following influenza virus infection are similar to those of humans (Belser et al. 2009).

It should be noted that 50% mice lethal dose (MLD_{50}) values, which are the most commonly used lethality indicator of H5N1 viruses, are highly variable from less than $10^{1.5}$ to more than 10^{7} depending on the strain (Lu et al. 1999; Katz et al. 2000b; Nguyen et al. 2005; Suguitan et al. 2006), suggesting that lethality of H5N1 virus is highly variable.

Recently, Kitajima et al. (2011) reported the development of time-dependent dose-response models for H5N1 virus based on survival data sets for experimental animals (mice or ferrets) exposed to graded doses of H5N1 virus.

In this study, a total of four candidate time-dependent dose-response models were fitted to four survival data sets, which were observed in different experimental conditions of hosts, virus strains, and inoculation routes, using the maximum-likelihood estimation.

Table 4. Data sets on infectivity of avian influenza A (H5N1) viruses in animal models

H5N1 virus strain[a]	Animal model[b]	ID_{50} [c]	k [d]	Reference
Isolates from humans				
HK/483/97	Mouse	$10^{0.5}$	2.2×10^{-1}	Nguyen et al. 2005
HK/483/97	Mouse	$10^{2.2}$	4.4×10^{-3}	Lu et al. 1999
HK/485/97	Mouse	$10^{1.1}$	5.5×10^{-2}	Lu et al. 1999
HK/156	Mouse	$10^{3.2}$	4.4×10^{-4}	Lu et al. 1999
HK/486	Mouse	$10^{1.2}$	4.4×10^{-2}	Lu et al. 1999
HK/483/97	Ferret	10^{2}	6.9×10^{-3}	Zitzow et al. 2002
HK/486	Ferret	10^{2}	6.9×10^{-3}	Zitzow et al. 2002
HK/213/03	Mouse	$10^{1.8}$	1.1×10^{-2}	Desheva et al. 2006
Thai/16/04	Mouse	$10^{1.3}$	3.5×10^{-2}	Maines et al. 2005
VN1203/04	Mouse	$10^{1.8}$	1.1×10^{-2}	Maines et al. 2005
VN1204/04	Mouse	$10^{2.3}$	3.5×10^{-3}	Maines et al. 2005
Thai/SP83/04	Mouse	$10^{1.8}$	1.1×10^{-2}	Maines et al. 2005
HK/213/03	Mouse	$10^{2.8}$	1.1×10^{-3}	Hoelscher et al. 2006
HK/483/97	Mouse	$10^{0.75}$	1.2×10^{-1}	Szretter et al. 2007
HK/486/97	Mouse	$10^{2.25}$	3.9×10^{-3}	Szretter et al. 2007
HK/483/97	Mouse	$10^{0.5}$	2.2×10^{-1}	Szretter et al. 2009
HK/486/97	Mouse	$10^{1.5}$	2.2×10^{-2}	Szretter et al. 2009
Isolates from birds				
Gs/VN/113/01	Mouse	$10^{4.3}$	3.5×10^{-5}	Nguyen et al. 2005
CK/Korea/ES/03	Mouse	$10^{1.8}$	1.1×10^{-2}	Lee et al. 2005
CK/Korea/ES/03	Mouse	$10^{2.3}$	3.5×10^{-3}	Maines et al. 2005
Ck/Indon/7/03	Mouse	$10^{5.3}$	3.5×10^{-6}	Maines et al. 2005
Ck/VN/NCVD8/03	Mouse	$10^{5.8}$	1.1×10^{-6}	Maines et al. 2005
Ck/VN/NCVD31/04	Mouse	$10^{3.5}$	2.2×10^{-4}	Maines et al. 2005
Dkmt/01	Mouse	$10^{4.5}$	2.2×10^{-5}	Lu et al. 1999

[a]All strains were *wild-type*; Multi-basic amino acid sequences, indicating high pathogenicity, were observed for all strains.

[b]Administrated intranasally to the model animals for all experiments.

[c]ID_{50}, 50% infectious dose; Values are expressed as 50% egg infectious dose (EID_{50}).

[d]Parameter of exponential dose-response model calculated by equation $k = -\frac{\ln 0.5}{ID_{50}}$.

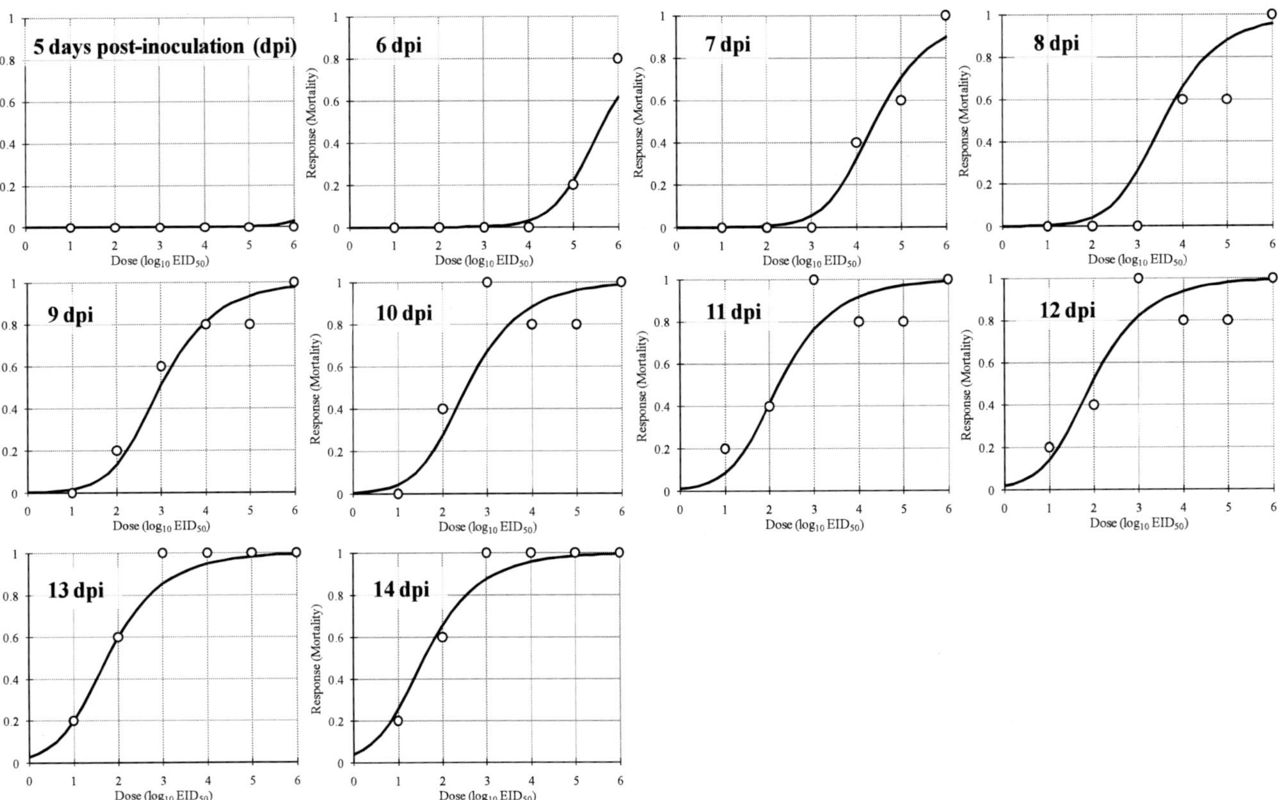

Figure 1. The best-fit model (beta-Poisson model with exponential-inverse-power DPI dependency) (curves) compared to observed mortalities against doses (symbols, Fan et al. 2009) (Kitajima et al. 2011).

It was demonstrated that a beta-Poisson dose-response model with the N_{50} parameter modified by an exponential-inverse-power time dependency or an exponential dose-response model with the k parameter modified by an exponential-inverse time dependency provided a statistically adequate fit to the observed survival data. As an example, Figure 1 shows the dose-response curve based on the best-fit model with the observed mortalities reported by Fan et al. (2009), and the best-fit time-dependent dose-response model is expressed as the following equation:

$$P(d) = 1 - [1 + \frac{d}{e^{(301.5/(DPI)^{1.793} + 1.000)}} \times (2^{\frac{1}{0.4640}} - 1)]^{-0.4640} \quad (7)$$

where, represents the probability of infection at the dose of d .

As shown in Figure 1, the best-fit model well predicted the observed responses. It was found that the best-fit model differed depending on the data set, probably due to the difference of host, virus strain, and/or inoculation route. The developed models were able to describe the mortality over time and represent observed experimental responses of mice or ferrets accurately. This is the first study describing time-dependent dose-response models for H5N1 virus (Kitajima et al. 2011). The models developed in this study, especially the models for ferrets that are excellent model to study human influenza virus infection, will be a useful tool for estimating the time-dependent mortality of H5N1 virus, for preparation of a future influenza pandemic caused by this lethal virus.

4. Prevention/Control of Waterborne Influenza Outbreaks

Sources of drinking water, surface water (such as reservoirs, rivers, and lakes), groundwater aquifers under influence of surface water, and rainwater collection systems may be susceptible to avian influenza virus contamination. Lénès et al. (2010) assessed the removal and inactivation of H5N1 and H1N1 viruses by water treatment processes. It was demonstrated that treatment plants designed to supply drinking water from surface water resources, which are generally composed of a coagulation-flocculation-settling process, a 1st stage filtration (sand filtration for example), an ozonation process, a 2nd stage filtration (granular activated carbon filtration for example), and a final disinfection, would readily be effective in removing and/or inactivating H5N1.

Since influenza viruses have an envelope that is susceptible to oxidizing agents including chlorine and ozone, they are considered to be relatively susceptible to disinfectants. Rice et al. (2007) demonstrated that H5N1 virus was readily inactivated by chlorination; the maintenance of a free chlorine residual (0.52-1.08 mg/L) was sufficient to inactivate the virus by >3 log within an exposure time of 1 minute.

When a proper pre-treatment process (e.g. coagulation, sedimentation and rapid sand filtration) to remove the chlorine demand associated with the treated water is performed, a chlorination process could achieve appreciable inactivation of influenza viruses and the water supplies are unlikely to pose a significant risk of infection even if infected waterfowl are present in source waters. It is important to ensure that chlorine or alternative disinfectant residuals is maintained throughout the water treatment and distribution systems; specifically, residual free chlorine of at least 0.5 mg/L after at least 30 min contact time at pH <8.0 should be maintained at a water treatment plant and residual chlorine concentration of 0.2 mg/L should be kept throughout the distribution system. Household-level interventions, such as home chlorination and boiling, are also effective at inactivating influenza viruses.

5. Future Study Directions

Pathogenesis and lethality of H5N1 virus is highly variable. In order to calculate infection risk and disease burden accurately, it is very important to understand the factors determining the transmissibility, infectivity, and lethality of H5N1 viruses. Hemagglutinin (HA) receptor specificity plays an important role in the transmission of influenza viruses and the affinity of viral HA protein for sialic acid-α2,6-galactose (SAα2,6-Gal; human-like receptors) is required for the transmission among ferrets which express SAα2,6-Gal on respiratory tract tissues. Recent finding revealed that four influenza virus proteins, not only HA but also PB2, NS1, and PB1-F2, are major determinants of virulence, pathogenicity, and host range restriction (Neumann et al. 2010). Although only a limited number of dose-response data on H5N1 virus are available to date, future dose-response analysis on H5N1 viruses should consider these molecular factors for better understanding of their pathogenesis and transmissibility among humans. Further QMRA works on H5N1 viruses should also include the application of the dose-response model by combining with the virus shedding, transportation, and exposure models, as described previously (Atkinson and Wein 2008; Nicas and Jones 2009).

CONCLUSION

Recently, information on the presence and stability of influenza viruses in water and sewage has been accumulated, although knowledge on H5N1 highly pathogenic virus is still lacking. Additional studies on the survival of the H5N1 virus in various types of water under field conditions would improve exposure assessment. Also, more information on the effective means for inactivation of the H5N1 virus in water and wastewater is needed. Accumulation of H5N1 virus-specific information will provide insights into the potential environmental risk factors and aid decision makers in prevention/control activities.

The QMRA framework can be a powerful tool to understand how to control pandemics mediated by environmental reservoirs or human-to-human transmission (e.g. calculating risk of infection due to a low dose). The recently developed QMRA models for H5N1 highly pathogenic avian influenza virus, such as the time-dependent dose-response models (Kitajima et al. 2011), will be useful to evaluate the risks of infection under various transmission scenarios and contribute to prevention of a future human influenza pandemic caused by this lethal virus.

REFERENCES

Armstrong, T. W. and C. N. Haas. 2007. A quantitative microbial risk assessment model for Legionnaires' disease: animal model selection and dose-response modeling. *Risk Anal.,* 27:1581–1596.

Atkinson, M. P., and L. M. Wein. 2008. Quantifying the routes of transmission for pandemic influenza. *Bull. Math. Biol.,* 70:820–867.

Bartrand, T. A., M. H. Weir, and C. N. Haas. 2008. Dose-response models for inhalation of Bacillus anthracis spores: interspecies comparisons. *Risk Anal.,* 28:1115–1124.

Belser, J. A., K. J. Szretter, J. M. Katz, and T. M. Tumpey. 2009. Use of animal models to understand the pandemic potential of highly pathogenic avian influenza viruses. *Adv. Virus Res.,* 73:55–97.

Brankston, G., Gitterman, L., Hirji, Z., Lemieux, C., Gardam, M. 2007. Transmission of influenza A in human beings. *Lancet Infect. Dis.,* 7:257-65.

Brown, J. D., D. E. Swayne, R, J. Cooper, R. E. Burns, and D. E. Stallknecht. 2007. Persistence of H5 and H7 avian influenza viruses in water. *Avian. Dis.,* 51(Suppl. 1):285-289.

Brown, J. D., Goekjian, G., Poulson, R., Valeika, S., Stallknecht, D. E. 2009. Avian influenza virus in water: infectivity is dependent on pH, salinity and temperature. *Vet. Microbiol.,* 136:20-26.

Buchy, P., S. Mardy, S. Vong, T. Toyoda, J. T. Aubin, M. Miller, S. Touch, L. Sovann, J. B. Dufourcq, B. Richner, P. V. Tu, N. T. Tien, W. Lim, J. S. Peiris, and S. Van der Werf. 2007. Influenza A/H5N1 virus infection in humans in Cambodia. *J. Clin. Virol.,* 39:164–168.

Chan, M. C., N. Lee, P. K. Chan, T. F. Leung, and J. J. Sung. 2009. Fecal detection of influenza A virus in patients with concurrent respiratory and gastrointestinal symptoms. *J. Clin. Virol.,* 45:208–211.

Deboosere N, Horm SV, Pinon A, Gachet J, Coldefy C, Buchy P, Vialette M. 2011. Development and validation of a concentration method for the detection of influenza a viruses from large volumes of surface water. *Appl. Environ. Microbiol.,* 77:3802-3808.

de Jong, M. D., V. C. Bach, T. Q. Phan, M. H. Vo, T. T. Tran, B. H. Nguyen, M. Beld, T. P. Le, H. K. Truong, V. V. Nguyen, T. H. Tran, Q. H. Do, and J. Farrar. 2005. Fatal avian influenza A (H5N1) in a child presenting with diarrhea followed by coma. *N. Engl. J. Med.,* 17:686–691.

Desheva, J. A., X. H. Lu, A. R. Rekstin, L. G. Rudenko, D. E. Swayne, N. J. Cox, J. M. Katz, and A. I. Klimov. 2006. Characterization of an influenza A H5N2 reassortant as a candidate for live-attenuated and inactivated vaccines against highly pathogenic H5N1 viruses with pandemic potential. *Vaccine,* 24:6859–6866.

Dovas, C. I., M. Papanastassopoulou, M. P. Georgiadis, E. Chatzinasiou, V. I. Maliogka, and G. K. Georgiades. 2010. Detection and quantification of infectious avian influenza A (H5N1) virus in environmental water by using real-time reverse transcription-PCR. *Appl. Environ. Microbiol.,* 76:2165-2174.

Dublineau A, Batéjat C, Pinon A, Burguière AM, Leclercq I, Manuguerra JC. 2011. Persistence of the 2009 pandemic influenza A (H1N1) virus in water and on non-porous surface. *PLoS One,* 6:e28043.

Fan, S., G. Deng, J. Song, G. Tian, Y. Suo, Y. Jiang, Y. Guan, Z. Bu, Y. Kawaoka, and H. Chen. 2009. Two amino acid residues in the matrix protein M1 contribute to the virulence difference of H5N1 avian influenza viruses in mice. *Virology,* 384:28–32.

Farrah SR, Gerba CP, Wallis C, Melnick JL. 1976. Concentration of viruses from large volumes of tap water using pleated membrane filters. *Appl. Environ. Microbiol.,* 31:221-226.

Haas, C.N. 1983. Estimation of risk due to low doses of microorganisms: a comparison of alternative methodologies. *Am. J. Epidemiol.,* 118: 573-582.

Haas, C. N., J. B. Rose, C. Gerba, and S. Regli. 1993. Risk assessment of virus in drinking water. *Risk Anal.,* 13:545–552.

Haas, C. N., J. B. Rose, and C. P. Gerba. 1999. Quantitative Microbial Risk Assessment. Wiley and Sons, New York, United States of America.

Haas, C. N., A. Thayyar-Madabusi, J. B. Rose, and C. P. Gerba. 2000. Development of a dose-response relationship for Escherichia coli O157:H7. *Int. J. Food Microbiol.,* 1:153–159.

Haramoto, E., H. Katayama, and S. Ohgaki. 2004. Detection of noroviruses in tap water in Japan by means of a new method for concentrating enteric viruses in large volumes of freshwater. *Appl. Environ. Microbiol.,* 70:2154–2160.

Heijnen L, Medema G. 2011. Surveillance of influenza A and the pandemic influenza A (H1N1) 2009 in sewage and surface water in the Netherlands. *J. Water Health,* 9:434-442.

Hénaux V, Samuel MD, Dusek RJ, Fleskes JP, Ip HS. 2012. Presence of avian influenza viruses in waterfowl and wetlands during summer 2010 in California: are resident birds a potential reservoir? *PLoS One,* 7:e31471.

Hinshaw VS, Webster RG, Turner B. 1979. Water-bone transmission of influenza A viruses? *Intervirology,* 11:66-68.

Hoelscher, M. A., S. Garg, D. S. Bangari, J. A. Belser, X. Lu, I. Stephenson, R. A. Bright, J. M. Katz, S. K. Mittal, and S. Sambhara. 2006. Development of adenoviral-vector-based pandemic influenza vaccine against antigenically distinct human H5N1 strains in mice. *Lancet,* 367:475–481.

Ito T, Okazaki K, Kawaoka Y, Takada A, Webster RG, Kida H. 1995. Perpetuation of influenza A viruses in Alaskan waterfowl reservoirs. *Arch. Virol.,* 140:1163-1172.

Katayama, H., A. Shimasaki, and S. Ohgaki. 2002. Development of a virus concentration method and its application to detection of enterovirus and Norwalk virus from coastal seawater. *Appl. Environ. Microbiol.,* 68:1033–1039.

Katz, J. M., X. Lu, A. M. Frace, T. Morken, S. R. Zaki, and T. M. Tumpey. 2000a. Pathogenesis of and immunity to avian influenza A H5 *viruses. Biomed. Pharmacother,* 54:178–187.

Katz, J. M., X. Lu, T. M. Tumpey, C. B. Smith, M. W. Shaw, and K. Subbarao. 2000b. Molecular correlates of influenza A H5N1 virus pathogenesis in mice. *J. Virol.,* 74:10807–10810.

de Jong, M.D. 2008. H5N1 transmission and disease: observations from the frontlines. *Pediatr. Infect. Dis. J.,* 27:S54–S56.

Khalenkov, A., W. G. Laver, and R. G. Webster. 2008. Detection and isolation of H5N1 influenza virus from large volumes of natural water. *J. Virol. Methods,* 149:180-183.

Kitajima M, Katayama H, Haas CN, Furumai H. 2010. Quantitative risk assessment of H5N1 highly pathogenic avian influenza virus infections through water. *Environmental Engineering Research,* 47:485-496. [In Japanese]

Kitajima M (2011) "Molecular epidemiological analysis of pathogenic viruses in water environments and risk assessment", Ph. D. dissertation, University of Tokyo.

Kitajima M, Huang Y, Watanabe T, Katayama H, Haas CN. 2011. Dose-response time modeling for highly pathogenic avian influenza A (H5N1) virus infection. *Lett. Appl. Microbiol.,* 53:438-444.

Lee, C. W., D. L. Suarez, T. M. Tumpey, H. W. Sung, Y. K. Kwon, Y. J. Lee, J. G. Choi, S. J. Joh, M. C. Kim, E. K. Lee, J. M. Park, X. Lu, J. M. Katz, E. Spackman, D. E. Swayne, and J. H. Kim. 2005. Characterization of highly pathogenic H5N1 avian influenza A viruses isolated from South Korea. *J. Virol.,* 79:3692–3702.

Lénès D, Deboosere N, Ménard-Szczebara F, Jossent J, Alexandre V, Machinal C, Vialette M. 2010. Assessment of the removal and inactivation of influenza viruses H5N1 and H1N1 by drinking water treatment. *Water Res.,* 44:2473-2486.

Lu, X., T. M. Tumpey, T. Morken, S. R. Zaki, N. J. Cox, and J. M. Katz. 1999. A mouse model for the evaluation of pathogenesis and immunity to influenza A (H5N1) viruses isolated from humans. *J. Virol.,* 73:5903–5911.

Neumann, G., H. Chen, G. F. Gao, Y. Shu, and Y. Kawaoka. 2010. H5N1 influenza viruses: outbreaks and biological properties. *Cell Res.,* 20:51–61.

Nicas, M., and R. M. Jones. 2009. Relative contributions of four exposure pathways to influenza infection risk. *Risk Anal.,* 29:1292–1303.

Nguyen, D.C., T. M. Uyeki, S. Jadhao, T. Maines, M. Shaw, Y. Matsuoka, C. Smith, T. Rowe, X. Lu, H. Hall, X. Xu, A. Balish, A. Klimov, T. M. Tumpey, D. E. Swayne, L. P. Huynh, H. K. Nghiem, H. H. Nguyen, and L. T. Hoang, N. J. Cox, and J. M. Katz. 2005. Isolation and characterization of avian influenza viruses, including highly pathogenic H5N1, from poultry in live bird markets in Hanoi, Vietnam, in 2001. *J. Virol.,* 79:4201–4212.

Maines, T. R., X. H. Lu, S. M. Erb, L. Edwards, J. Guarner, P. W. Greer, D. C. Nguyen, K. J. Szretter, L. M. Chen, P. Thawatsupha, M. Chittaganpitch, S. Waicharoen, D. T. Nguyen, T. Nguyen, H. H. Nguyen, J. H. Kim, L. T. Hoang, C. Kang, L. S. Phuong, W. Lim, S. Zaki, R. O. Donis, N. J. Cox, J. M. Katz, and T. M. Tumpey. 2005. Avian influenza (H5N1) viruses isolated from humans in Asia in 2004 exhibit increased virulence in mammals. *J. Virol.,* 79:11788–11800.

Quantitative Microbial Risk Assessment (QMRA) Wiki, available at: http://wiki.camra.msu.edu/index.php?title=Quantitative_Microbial_Risk_Assessment_(QMRA)_Wiki, accessed on September 04, 2012.

Rice EW, Adcock NJ, Sivaganesan M, Brown JD, Stallknecht DE, Swayne DE. 2007. Chlorine inactivation of highly pathogenic avian influenza virus (H5N1). *Emerg. Infect. Dis.,* 13:1568-1570.

Roepke DC, Halvorson DA, Goyal SM, Kelleher CJ. 1989. An adsorption-elution technique for the recovery of influenza virus from water. *Avian. Dis.,* 33:649-653.

Schijven, J. F., P. F. M. Teunis, and A. M. de Roda Husman. 2005a. Quantitative risk assessment of avian influenza virus infection via water. *RIVM report,* 70319012.

Sivanandan V, Halvorson DA, Laudert E, Senne DA, Kumar MC. 1991. Isolation of H13N2 influenza A virus from turkeys and surface water. *Avian. Dis.,* 35:974-947.

Spackman E, Senne DA, Myers TJ, Bulaga LL, Garber LP, Perdue ML, Lohman K, Daum LT, Suarez DL. 2002. Development of a real-time reverse transcriptase PCR assay for type A influenza virus and the avian H5 and H7 hemagglutinin subtypes. *J. Clin. Microbiol.,* 40:3256-3260.

Stallknecht DE, Shane SM, Kearney MT, Zwank PJ. 1990a. Persistence of avian influenza viruses in water. *Avian. Dis.,* 34:406-411.

Stallknecht DE, Kearney MT, Shane SM, Zwank PJ. 1990b. Effects of pH, temperature, and salinity on persistence of avian influenza viruses in water. *Avian. Dis.,* 34:412-418.

Stone B, Burrows J, Schepetiuk S, Higgins G, Hampson A, Shaw R, Kok T. 2004. Rapid detection and simultaneous subtype differentiation of influenza A viruses by real time PCR. *J. Virol. Methods,* 117:103-112.

Suguitan, A. L. Jr., J. McAuliffe, K. L. Mills, H. Jin, G. Duke, B. Lu, C. J. Luke, B. Murphy, D.E. Swayne, G. Kemble, and K. Subbarao. 2006. Live, attenuated influenza A H5N1 candidate vaccines provide broad cross-protection in mice and ferrets. *PLoS Med.,* 73:5903–5911.

Szretter, K. J., S. Gangappa, X. Lu, C. Smith, W. J. Shieh, S. R. Zaki, S. Sambhara, T. M. Tumpey, and J. M. Katz. 2007. Role of host cytokine responses in the pathogenesis of avian H5N1 influenza viruses in mice. *J. Virol.,* 81:2736–2744.

Szretter, K. J., S. Gangappa, J. A. Belser, H. Zeng, H. Chen, Y. Matsuoka, S. Sambhara, D. E. Swayne, T. M. Tumpey, and J. M. Katz. 2009. Early control of H5N1 influenza virus replication by the type I interferon response in mice. *J. Virol.,* 83:5825–5834.

Teunis, P. F., C. L. Chappell, and P. C. Okhuysen. 2002. *Cryptosporidium* dose response studies: variation between isolates. *Risk Anal.,* 22:175–183.

To K. K., K. H. Chan, I. W. Li, T. Y. Tsang, H. Tse, J. F. Chan, I. F. Hung, S. T. Lai, C. W. Leung, Y. W. Kwan, Y. L. Lau, T. K. Ng, V. C. Cheng, J .S. Peiris, and K. Y. Yuen. 2010. Viral load in patients infected with pandemic H1N1 2009 influenza A virus. *J. Med. Virol.,* 82:1–7.

Vong S, Ly S, Van Kerkhove MD, Achenbach J, Holl D, Buchy P, Sorn S, Seng H, Uyeki TM, Sok T, Katz JM. 2009. Risk factors associated with subclinical human infection with avian influenza A (H5N1) virus--Cambodia, 2006. *J. Infect. Dis.,* 199:1744-1752.

Watanabe, T., T. A. Bartrand, M. H. Weir, T. Omura, and C. N. Haas. 2010. Development of a dose-response model for SARS coronavirus. *Risk Anal.,* 30:1129–1138.

Watanabe T, Bartrand TA, Omura T, Haas CN. Dose-Response Assessment for Influenza A Virus Based on Data Sets of Infection with its Live Attenuated Reassortants. *Risk Anal.,* 32:555–565.

Webster RG, Bean WJ, Gorman OT, Chambers TM, Kawaoka Y. 1992. Evolution and ecology of influenza A viruses. *Microbiol. Rev.,* 56:152-179.

Webster, R. G., M. Yakhno, V. S. Hinshaw, W. J. Bean, and K. G. Murti. 1978. Intestinal influenza: replication and characterization of influenza viruses in ducks. *Virology,* 84:268-278.

Wootton, S. H., D. W. Scheifele, A. Mak, M. Petric, and D. M. Skowronski. 2006. Detection of human influenza virus in the stool of children. *Pediatr. Infect. Dis. J.,* 25:1194–1195.

Wright, P.F., Neumann, G. and Kawaoka Y. (2007) Orthomyxoviruses. In Fields Virology ed. Knipe, D. and Howley, P. pp. 949–979. Philadelphia: Lippincott Williams and Wilkins.

Yoo SJ, Moon SJ, Kuak EY, Yoo HM, Kim CK, Chey MJ, Shin BM. 2010. Frequent detection of pandemic (H1N1) 2009 virus in stools of hospitalized patients. *J. Clin. Microbiol.,* 48:2314-2315.

Zhang G, Shoham D, Gilichinsky D, Davydov S, Castello JD, Rogers SO. 2006. Evidence of influenza a virus RNA in siberian lake ice. *J. Virol.,* 80:12229-12235.

Zhang H, Xu B, Chen Q, Chen J, Chen Z. 2011. Characterization of an H10N8 influenza virus isolated from Dongting lake wetland. *Virol. J.,* 8:42.

Zitzow, L.A., T. Rowe, T. Morken, W. J. Shieh, S. Zaki, and J. M. Katz. 2002. Pathogenesis of avian influenza A (H5N1) viruses in ferrets. *J. Virol.,* 76:4420–4429.

In: Avian Influenza
Editors: K. M. Taylor and B. O'Connor ISBN: 978-1-62417-415-5

Chapter 2

BIOSECURITY MEASURES AGAINST HIGHLY PATHOGENIC AVIAN INFLUENZA (HPAI) IN FREE-RANGE FLOCKS AND COMMERCIAL POULTRY IN DEVELOPING COUNTRIES: A REVIEW

Nma Bida Alhaji[1]* ***and Ismail Ayoade Odetokun***[2]

[1]State Veterinary Hospital,
Niger State Ministry of Livestock and Fisheries Development,
Bosso, Minna, Nigeria
[2]Department Veterinary Public Health and Preventive Medicine,
University of Ibadan, Ibadan, Nigeria

ABSTRACT

The emerging and re-emerging of infectious diseases over the last few decades demonstrate the potential for introduction of epidemic illnesses such as avian influenza through global migration of animals and humans. Recent outbreaks of a highly pathogenic avian influenza (HPAI) strain H5N1 in Asia and Africa have caused severe impacts on the poultry industries worldwide, both through bird mortality and morbidity and the resultant trade restrictions and negative demand shocks. There is also a

* Correspondence: N. B. Alhaji., Tel.: +234 (0)803 595 0915, E-mail: nmabida62@yahoo.com.

considerable global concern that the virus could mutate into a form that can be passed between humans, which poses a significant risk of leading to a global pandemic. The risk 'mitigation' measures and risk 'propagation' practices in free-range flocks could influence introduction and maintenance of low pathogenic avian influenza (LPAI) with consequent depression in immunity of the free-range flocks, mutation and development of HPAI. These enormous potential liabilities have led to significant global investments in the disease prevention and control. However, poultry producers have roles to play in the prevention and control of avian influenza.

In this study, we review biosecurity measures practice in free-range flocks and commercial poultry operations in developing countries. The scientific literature on the prevention/control of highly pathogenic avian influenza of the past years is reviewed. The review findings are plausible as birds from free-range flocks have more opportunities of contact with wild birds that serve as reservoirs of low-pathogenic avian influenza strains than the commercial poultry, thus providing them with constant challenge of flock immunity. The development of efficient and effective biosecurity measures against avian influenza on commercial farms requires adequate placements of barriers to provide segregation, cleaning and disinfection, while concerted community established sanitary measures are needed for free-range poultry flocks in the developing economies. Good biosecurity levels on the farms and in the flocks ultimately lower costs in the production cycle, and flock welfare is always enhanced.

Keywords: Highly pathogenic avian influenza (HPAI), free-range flocks, commercial poultry biosecurity

Introduction

The emerging and re-emerging of infectious diseases over the last few decades demonstrate the potential for introduction of epidemic illnesses such as avian influenza through global migration of animals and humans. Recent outbreaks of a highly pathogenic avian influenza (HPAI) strain H5N1 in Asia and Africa have caused severe impacts on the poultry industries worldwide, both through bird mortality and morbidity and the resultant trade restrictions and negative demand shocks. There is also a considerable global concern that the virus could mutate into a form that can be passed between humans, which poses a significant risk of leading to a global pandemic. Since late 2003, more than 150 million birds have been culled in attempts to stem the spread of the

Asian lineage of H5N1 in domestic flocks, but this has not prevented the further spread of the virus – although it has helped reduce the threat in certain regions and countries [1]. Avian influenza has been listed by the World Organization for Animal Health (OIE) as a disease of great importance to both human and animal health, listed under the Terrestrial Animal Health Code (Article 10.4) as a Notifiable Avian Influenza (NAI). One of the reasons for this listing is mainly due to the high social and economic consequences and constant threat to public health resulting from outbreaks. Trade and movement of poultry and poultry products have been associated with the spread of the disease across Nigeria [2, 3].

Globalization and relative ease of transportation has caused an expansion of infection zone of avian influenza. Impacts on the poultry industries worldwide both through bird mortality and morbidity have been seen. Poultry serve as an important resource to the livelihoods of the poor and underprivileged providing food (egg and meat), income and household necessities. Apart from avian influenza causing great losses in world economies owing to death of affected birds, serious illnesses, death, social disruption and economic losses are seen among the human populace in various regions [4]. An average percentage (57%) of poultry workers is aware that avian influenza has food safety implications [5]. After the 2006 HPAI H5N1 outbreak in Nigeria, negative economic and nutritional effects were noticed and over 770,000 birds died due to disease [6]. Village poultry especially those raised on free range and which are very important to the livelihoods of many local communities were seriously affected. These enormous potential liabilities have led to significant global investments in the disease prevention and control. Stakeholders in the poultry industry have significant roles to play in the prevention and control of avian influenza.

Avian Influenza Outbreaks of Concern in Developing Countries

Various reports on the three very important influenza pandemics that occurred during the 20th century abound in literatures. The Spanish flu (H1N1) of 1918-1919 was noted for its high transmission and severity, causing approximately 40 million deaths worldwide. The Asian flu (H2N2) of 1957-58 was characterized with severe episodes worldwide, with children most affected [7]. By 1958, about 4 million people were lost to this outbreak [8]. Hong Kong flu (H3N2) of 1968-69 was the third major influenza pandemic with about 2 million deaths [8]. It also had a wide distribution with occurrences in the UK and US. In 2003, there was an unexpected outbreak of avian influenza and it was officially reported as the highly pathogenic avian influenza (HPAI) H5N1 in four Asian countries, with the second wave (the resurgent) reported between mid-2004 and 2005. The third wave of occurrence which has now become global and endemic in some specific countries in Asia and Africa started in mid 2005 [9]. Consequently, high numbers of birds and human morbidities have been recorded because of its ability to spread rapidly across international borders at an alarming rate, endemicity of Asia, Africa and other developing countries, with high mutation and morbidity and mortality rates [7].

Highly pathogenic avian influenza virus H5N1 was first officially reported in Africa in early 2006 in Nigeria [10, 11, 12, 13]. In Nigeria, HPAI H5N1 outbreaks have not been reported in the free-range flocks [14]. After its first emergence in Nigeria, other outbreaks have been recorded in over 10 African countries such as Niger, Cameroon, Egypt, Sudan, Burkina Faso, Djibouti, Ivory Coast, Ghana, Togo, and Benin [15]. HPAI H5N1 spread fast across international borders at an alarming rate making the world to be at a high risk of a possible pandemic in the nearest future [7]. A continuing danger of resurging HPAI outbreaks exists in smallholder farming systems, where the disease is more difficult to control. There are also concerns that some genotypes of HPAI H5N1 strains might have adapted to backyard indigenous terrestrial poultry in the same way they have to domestic ducks, thus sustaining the risk of further outbreaks and mutations [14].

Risk Factors Facilitating The Spread of Avian Influenza in Poultry

The highly pathogenic avian influenza (HPAI) H5N1 virus has spread across Eurasia into Africa. Its persistence in a number of countries continues to disrupt poultry production, impairs smallholder livelihoods, and raises the risk that a genotype adapted to human-to-human transmission may emerge from it. While domestic ducks have been identified as reservoirs and primary risk factor associated with HPAI H5N1 persistence in poultry in Southeast Asia, little is known of such factors in countries with different agro-ecological conditions such as Nigeria. However, environment can play vital role in the propagation of the virus [16]. Of important risk in the spread of HPAI is the relatedness of AI viruses isolated in Africa to those existing across the globe especially in the Asian countries. A phylogenic analysis carried out on some AI strains isolated from birds across Africa discovered an appreciable level of relatedness with HPAI H5N1 viruses circulating across the length and breadth of Europe and the Middle East [15]. Another plausible finding was the discovery of genes with mutational characteristics encoded for host adaptations and high resistance to antiviral agents in human influenza viruses in the bird isolates. This raises a concern of public health importance. Similarly, full-length genomic sequences of HPAI H5N1 isolates from Nigeria and Burkina Faso had shown African isolates to be clustered within three sub-lineages with distinct nucleotide and amino acid signatures and geographical distribution in

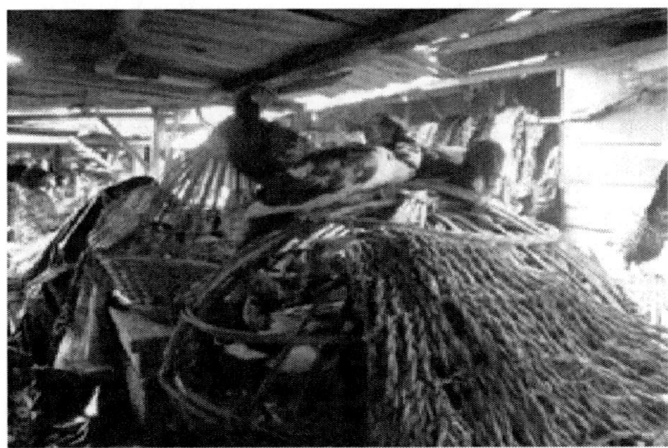

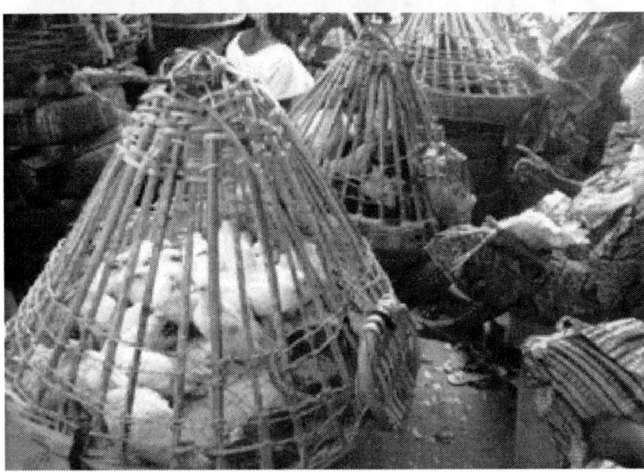

Figure 1. (Continued).

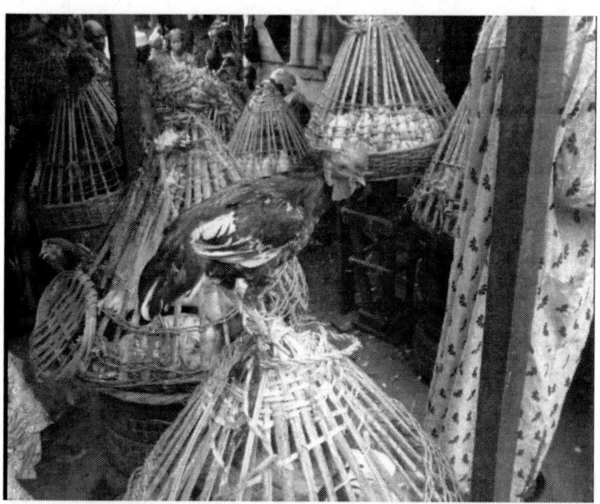

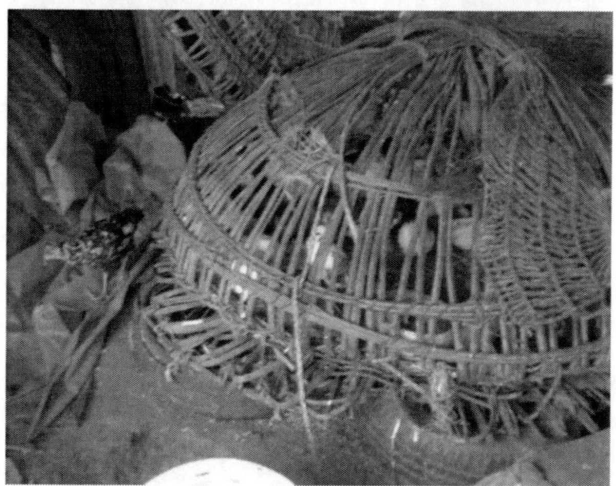

Figure 1. Interspecies mixing of birds at live bird markets (LBMs) in developing country.

Africa. Some isolates were traced to have entered Africa through the East African/West Asian and Black Sea/Mediterranean flyways of migratory birds [17]. The reason for this is largely due to high level of interaction among migratory birds, water birds and the commercially raised poultry or free ranged flocks. The sub-Saharan Africa over the years have served and still serving as a shelter for large number of Eurasian birds after seasonal migrations [18]. In a surveillance of avian influenza in wild birds across Africa, LPAI were detected in several species of wild birds in both West and

East Africa which translates to the fact that this virus thrives successfully under the environmental conditions of the afro-tropical ecosystem and avian influenza viruses remain in these birds throughout the year [19]. A major contributory risk identified is the movement and international travels involving both human and animal components. The main factors in small-scale commercial farms in Africa may be due to uncontrolled livestock and poultry movement within and outside the continent owing to the lack of enforcement of animal disease control laws and regulation in most of the countries, including registration and licensing of poultry farms and hatcheries. Increased close contact between poultry and human, and lack of organized poultry marketing that encourages open live poultry markets and interspecies mixing and poor sanitary conditions could be responsible for the high risks among free-range and backyard poultry flocks [14, 20, 21].

The high risks of avian influenza virus occurrence and propagation are also mostly associated with sources of water and feed, poor handling of litter, drinkers, feeders and environment which could create favorable conditions for introduction and mutation of low pathogenic avian influenza (LPAI) to HPAI. However, the high risks for commercial poultry farms is a combination of risk 'mitigation' (isolation of birds to confinement) and risk 'propagation' (traffic into the farm with feed) measures [14, 22]. The risk 'mitigation' measures and risk 'propagation' practices in free-range flocks could influence introduction and maintenance of low pathogenic avian influenza (LPAI) with consequent depression in immunity of the free-range flocks, mutation and development of HPAI. These enormous potential liabilities have led to significant global investments in the disease prevention and control.

A number of common practices in animal husbandry can also be risk factors facilitating the spread/transmission of virus between domestic free range flock and wild birds. These include location of poultry operations in migratory wild bird flyways; open access to watering and feeding areas by migratory wild birds and domestic poultry; and waste runoffs from domestic poultry operations that end up in wetlands used by migratory wild birds. Furthermore, the inadequate or low quality of vaccines use in poultry operations might provide "cover" for the emergence of pathogenic avian influenza viral strains in domestic fowl. The viral agents themselves may encourage resistant or mutant strains, such as from low pathogenic to highly strains. Using a traffic light system model developed by [23] in determining the HPAI risks in small-scale commercial farms, high risks levels were noticed to be apparently increasing the vulnerability of the farms to HPAI infection such that favorable conditions for introduction and mutation of LPAI could be established [14]. These farms operate confined management system with minimal biosecurity, associated sources of water and feed, poor handling of litter, drinkers, feeders and environment.

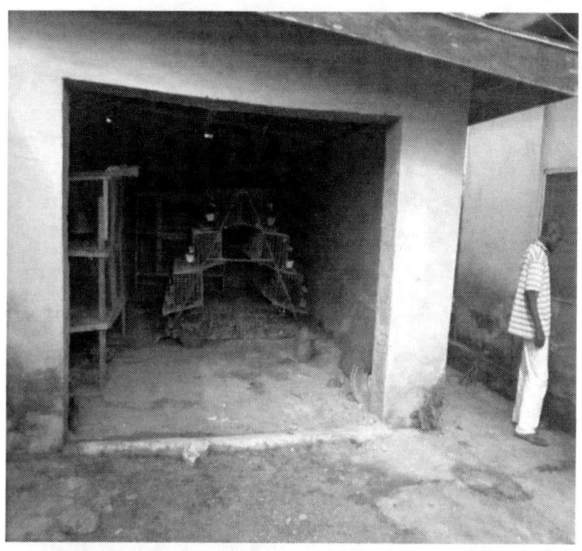

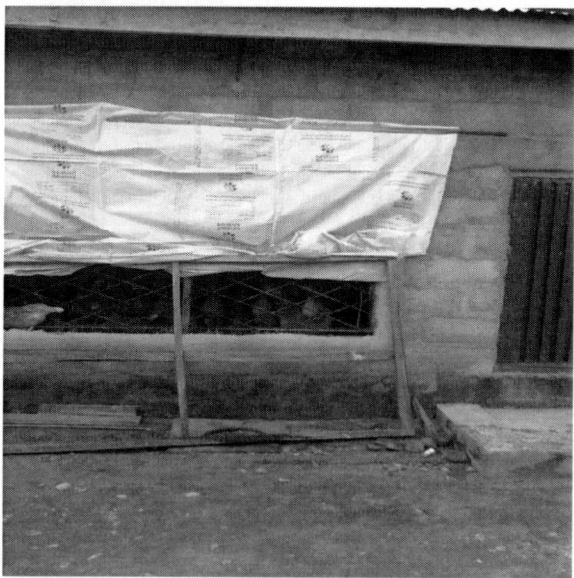

Figure 2. (Continued).

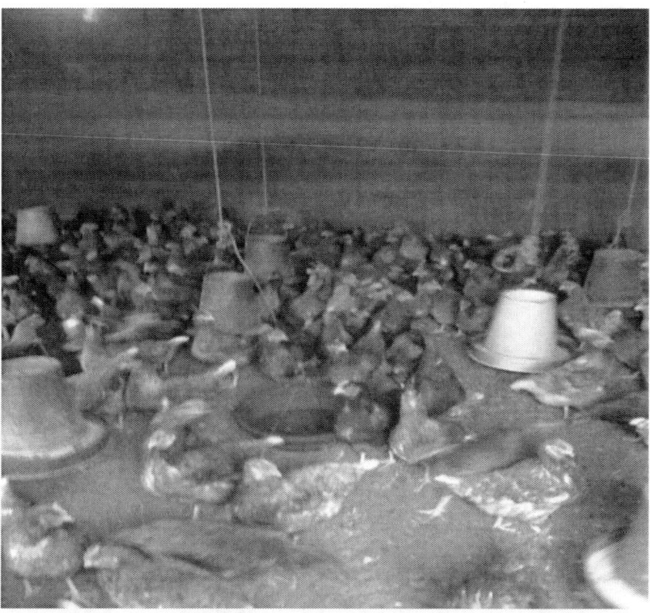

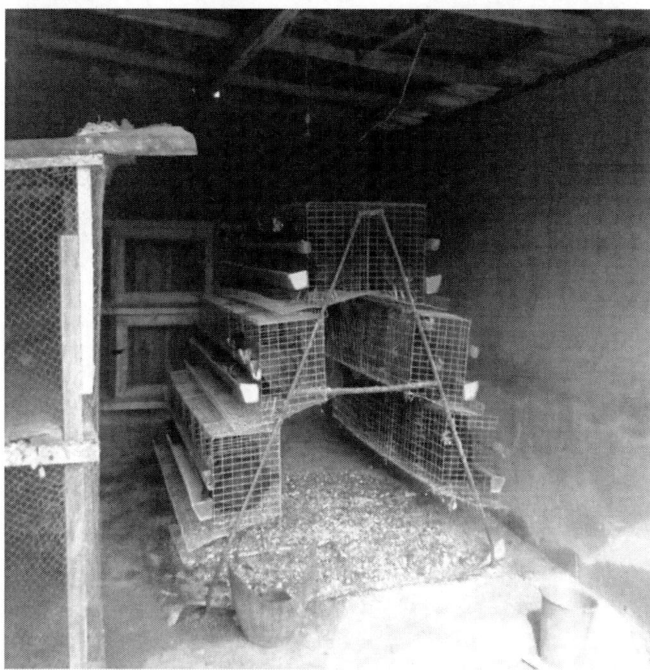

Figure 2. Backyard poultry farm in developing country.

This is congruent to documented occurrence in Thailand [22]. The free range flocks are at lower risk of HPAI H5N1 infections compared to small-scale commercial operations [14, 22]. Possible reasons for the low risk levels in backyard flocks may be due to continuous exposure to LPAI while HPAI requires favorable ecological and landscape factors such as presence of wetlands, high flock stock density; confinement, waste presence and poor ventilation to facilitate transmission between wild birds and domestic flocks [22, 24, 25, 26].

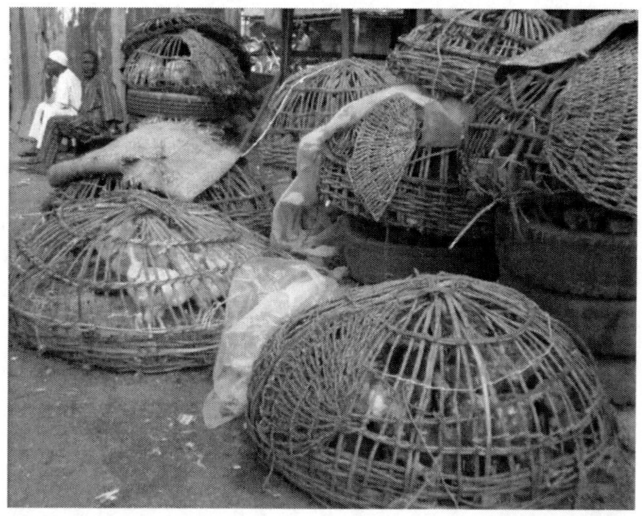

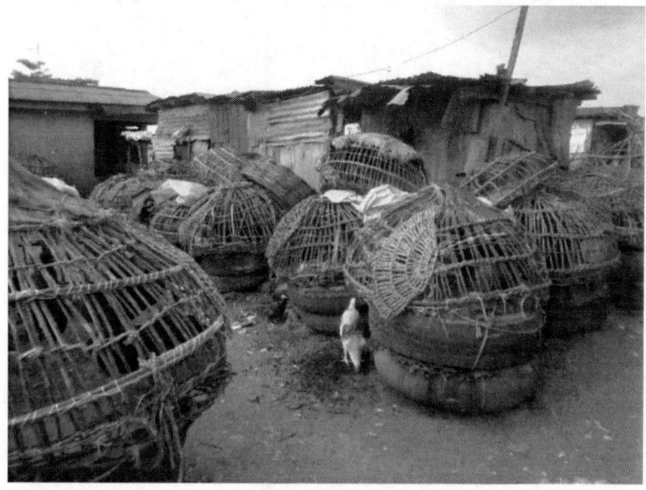

Figure 3. (Continued).

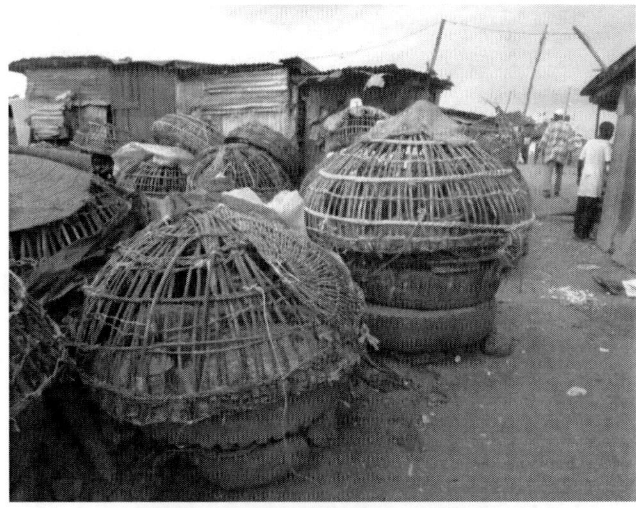

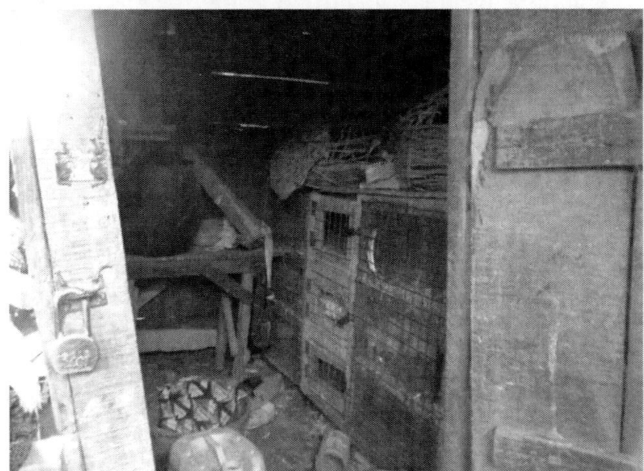

Figure 3. Poor sanitation in LBMs, a biosecurity challenge in developing country.

The exposed free-range flocks have more opportunities to contact wild bird reservoirs of LPAI strains than small-scale commercial poultry, thus providing them with constant challenge and maintenance of flock immunity [14]. Thus, both wild birds and free-range flocks could serve as potential source of HPAI for commercial birds when contact is facilitated. HPAI viruses primarily infect poultry in which viruses of subtypes H5 and H7, presumably from wild birds or contact with their derivatives, sporadically switch to highly virulent strains [27]. Between 1999 and 2000, a severe avian influenza (H7N1) known to have evolved from a LPAI caused an epidemic in Italy affecting commercial, game and back-yard flocks [28]. There are now strong indications that genotypes of H5N1 strains have adapted to backyard, indigenous terrestrial poultry akin to way they have in domestic ducks, hence further sustaining the risk of outbreaks and mutations [9].

CONTROL OF HPAI IN DEVELOPING COUNTRIES

Biosecurity Measures

Deaths of poultry flocks resulting from the HPAI H5N1 virus in developing countries, most especially in Africa since 2006 have been very alarming. Occurrences in Burkina Faso, Cameroon, Djibouti, Egypt, Ivory Coast, Niger, Nigeria and Sudan identified initially were localized to the area of their first introduction but those noticed in Egypt and Nigeria were more refractory covering the lengths and breadths of the countries. The outbreaks spread fast becoming multi-state and national problems. Considering the potential effect of influenza pandemic on the public health, national, regional and international economies, it is important that necessary steps be taken as a priority to prevent and control this disease. It is also critical that appropriate arrangements are made for its early detection and control. Poultry producers have roles to play in the prevention and control of avian influenza in both free range flocks and commercial poultry farms. Biosecurity is the most essential procedure in the prevention and control of the HPAI. Its application should be the initial step in checking the introduction of avian influenza into farms and poultry flocks [29, 30, 31] and in the event of an initial spread of avian influenza among birds, biosecurity is one of the key pillars in slowing the spread [32].

Biosecurity is the implementation of measures that reduce the risk of the introduction and spread of disease agents; it requires the adoption of a set of attitudes and behaviors by people to reduce risk in all activities involving domestic, exotic and wild birds and their products [32]. Biosecurity is broadly based on two viable principles of bio-containment and bio-exclusion. All actions taken to prevent the introduction of infectious agents into flocks and premises are termed bio-exclusion while bio-containment involves limiting the spread of the virus within the flock/farm and not allowing the infection to spread outside the farm. For a thorough and effective prevention of the incursion of HPAI in developing countries, strong biosecurity defense line should be instituted in large and small scale commercial poultry producers, hatcheries, free-range birds, live bird markets (LBMs), intermediaries and service providers, poultry fanciers, and keepers of fighting cocks, exotic birds and birds of prey and hunters [32]. The risk factors and status of biosecurity measures against HPAI in Nigeria signifies variations in poultry production system across the country [14]. The inability of the local poultry farms and free range flocks in Nigeria to attain a low risk status signifies inadequate sanitary efforts to effect risk reduction in HPAI and other infectious poultry diseases. The development of efficient and effective biosecurity measures against poultry diseases on small-scale commercial farms requires adequate placement of barriers to provide segregation, cleaning and disinfection [14]. The awareness level of poultry attendants is an important tool in controlling the spread of HPAI. Over 50% of sampled attendants in infected poultry farms with the HPAI were aware of threats linked with processing of HPAI-infected chicken meat, with the awareness level higher in workers of urban/peri-urban than rural centers. Consequently, rural livestock raisers may be at a high risk of human-avian influenza virus contact due to the discrepancies in the awareness levels [5].

This cannot be compared with the situation in some Asian countries such as China and Thailand. For instance in China, the awareness level is high among both in urban and rural dwellers on avian influenza [33]. Some identified factors negating biosecurity in many developing countries include close and direct contact of infected birds with healthy ones, home slaughtering, unprotected personnel, eating and processing of infected carcasses, inadequate use of disinfectants, and visits to markets. This indicates that the knowledge and awareness level of poultry workers is an important component of biosecurity against HPAI spread and outbreaks. Good biosecurity levels act as a preventive measure for birds on the farms and in the flocks ultimately lower costs in the production cycle, and therefore flock welfare is always enhanced. To effectively prevent outbreaks of HPAI H5N1 in developing countries, there is a need for rehabilitation and revitalization of exiting veterinary quarantine infrastructure and personnel to ensure adequate and constant poultry disease surveillance and developing reliable mechanisms for strict monitoring of movement of poultry and products. Veterinary facilities available in most developing countries (for instance, Nigeria) do not meet OIE standards, while the ratio of the existing facilities to poultry farms and flocks range from 1:500 in rural areas to 1: 400 in urban areas [34]. There should be shift of attention to commercial poultry farms and hatcheries and much paid on free-range/backyard poultry farms. Community based enlightenment and training of free-range poultry farmers on specific biosecurity procedures, HPAI clinical signs recognition in birds and control under local settings need to be instituted with encouragement of regional and international cooperation for HPAI H5N1 prevention and control. Existing Live bird markets (LBMs) with interspecies mixing of birds should be reorganized while close interactions between humans and birds should be reduced. In event of outbreaks, stamping out should be immediately instituted with full compensation for livestock/flock owners whose birds are slaughtered. Affected and slaughtered flocks should be properly disposed. Sale and consumption of sick and dead birds should also be discouraged.

Cleaning and Disinfection

Cleaning is one of the most effective ways of preventing the spread of HPAI. Poultry houses and surroundings as well as all equipments used in various management operations must be systematically cleaned as this would aid disinfection. Poultry houses should be cleaned from back to front and top to bottom. Usually, disinfectants are more effective on cleaned and wet surfaces. Cleaning is almost nil among free-range poultry operators in Africa. Control of animal diseases is usually enhanced by use of disinfectants when decontaminating the farm environment. Some poultry farms in Nigeria do not use the right disinfectants at appropriate concentrations in disinfection. In a survey carried out in North central Nigeria, only 56% of commercial poultry raisers clean the equipments they use with disinfectant while those that raise birds on free-range rarely use disinfectants and sanitizers [14]. This is the situation in most rural and sub-urban poultry farms in Africa. Disinfection has been identified as a veritable tool in the prevention of H5N1 virus infection in poultry establishments.

Disinfectants such as sodium hypochlorite, 70% ethanol, oxidizing agents, quaternary ammonium compounds, aldehydes (formalin, glutaraldehyde, and formaldehyde), phenols, acids, povidone-iodine and lipid solvents can inactivate influenza viruses when used appropriately [35]. These agents are effective at varying temperatures and pH [36]. Chlorine is regarded as the best disinfectant against avian influenza (H5N1) viruses [37]. Some workers (21%) in Nigeria believed that thorough cleaning, cooking (including traditional) and frying methods were adequate to HPAI virus present in poultry foods (chicken and eggs) sourced from HPAI infected farms [5]. The virus persists in the environment thereby underscoring the need for regular disinfection of poultry premises [38]. Analyses of viral genetic sequences from recent H5N1 outbreaks in Thailand support the concept that viruses re-emerge from a small pool of indigenous sources where they survive the inter-outbreak season and are silently perpetuated over the dry summer months. Results suggest that eradication of H5N1 avian influenza could be accomplished by eliminating the local reservoirs [39].

Bio-Exclusion: Enhanced Biosecurity

Traditionally this practice takes place at the farm level and the best way to prevent HPAI from spreading through prevention of exposure of flocks to the influenza virus. This depends on the formation of a barrier between farms and the outside environment. Although this approach is still considered the cornerstone for prevention, recent experience has shown that maintaining high biosecurity standards to prevent spread is challenging. Strategies to enhance biosecurity in the poultry farms have been developed and involve the following [40]:

1) Avoid contact between domestic poultry and wild birds, especially waterfowl.
2) Avoid introduction of birds of unknown disease status into a flock.
3) Control human traffic. Ensure that people with access to the flock wear proper safety equipment such as boots, coveralls, gloves, face masks, and headgear. Provide clean clothing and disinfection facilities for employees.
4) Follow proper cleaning and disinfection procedures.
5) Use an "all-in/all-out" production system.
6) Permit only essential workers and vehicles to enter the farm.
7) Thoroughly clean and disinfect equipment and vehicles entering and leaving the farm; the tires and undercarriage of vehicles should be included in the process.
8) Do not loan or borrow equipment or vehicles from other farms.
9) Avoid visiting other poultry farms. If unavoidable or if visiting a live-bird market, change footwear and clothing before working with your own flock
10) Do not bring birds from slaughter channels, especially live-bird markets, back to the farm.

Bio-Containment: Outbreak Control in Poultry

These are steps put in place to control outbreak of HPAI [40]:

1) Controlled movement of birds and products that may contain virus Infected "zones" should be identified and movement of items and birds from those zones should be controlled. Border controls should be instituted as necessary.
   Destruction of infected and at-risk poultry ("stamping out"). This should be done within 24 hours after infection in the flock is detected and as humanely and as quickly as possible. One widely used method is asphyxiation using carbon dioxide. Stringent cleaning and disinfection of the facilities and equipment should be performed after culling. No new birds should be allowed in facilities for at least 21 days after depopulation and disinfection.
2) Proper disposal of carcasses and all animal products in contact with the infected flock should be performed in a biosecured and environmentally acceptable manner.
3) Vaccination of flocks may be suitable for control in some situations or may be used as an adjunct to mass culling efforts [29].

Live Markets

Once there is an outbreak of avian influenza virus in a live market, it can easily spread to other farms and/or markets via movement of birds, crates, or trucks. It is important to follow biosecurity protocols at live-bird markets as well as on the farm [40]. These protocols are:

1) Use plastic instead of wooden crates for easier cleaning.
2) Keep scales and floors clean of manure, feathers, and other debris.
3) Clean and disinfect all equipment, crates, and vehicles before returning them to the farm.
4) Keep incoming poultry separate from unsold birds, especially if birds are from different farms.
5) Clean and disinfect the marketplace after every day of sale.
6) Do not return unsold birds to the farm.

Vaccination

Until recently, avian influenza infections caused by viruses of the H5 and H7 subtype occurred rarely, and vaccination was not considered because stamping out was the recommended control option [29]. Vaccinated birds are less likely to become infected and are less likely to excrete the virus. Although vaccination has not been in conventional practice in Nigeria and some African countries, it can be used both as a tool to support eradication or as control the disease and reduce the viral load in the environment. There are three broad categories of vaccination strategies [40]:

1) Vaccination in response to an outbreak using a "ring vaccination" approach or vaccination of only designated high-risk poultry. This approach should be used in conjunction with culling of infected poultry.
2) Vaccination in response to a "trigger," such as evidence from active surveillance that a HPAI virus has detected in an area. This approach may be used in situations where the potential to improve biosecurity is limited.
3) Preemptive baseline vaccination, such as vaccinating poultry during restocking of farms in previously infected areas.

Basic Commercial Farm Biosecurity Measures

The high stock density of commercial farms in developing countries requires preventive biosecurity protocols. Preventive biosecurity measures instituted in commercial flocks should include:

1) Designing and building farm structures in appropriate layouts that would allow proper ventilation of farm premises.
2) Poultry houses should be well built with durable material and also designed for preventing influx of insects and pests. The farm area should be well delineated and well-fenced. This will limit movement of wild birds and carriers of HPAI into farms. Insects and pests should be regularly controlled using appropriate insecticides, pesticides and more preventively their barriers.
3) The services of veterinary experts and other animal health professionals should be employed in the management of poultry diseases.

4) Farming operations should be separated. Dirty and clean operations on the farm should be unconnected.
5) Farms workers should be enlightened on various biosecurity measures that should be instituted in preventing the introduction and spread of HPAI in farms.
6) The numbers of poultry workers should be limited while their movement should be restricted from pen to pen. There should be use of separate overalls and change of outdoors shoes before entering the flock houses. Feet dips should be provided in all entrance and should be habitually cleaned and disinfecting solutions must be changed regularly.
7) Any vehicle coming and leaving the farm premises (clothing, tools and equipment such as cages, bicycle, motorcycles and automobile tires) must be cleaned and disinfected.
8) Relationship with other farms and farm owners/workers should be restricted. Equipment and vehicles should not be borrowed from other farms. Birds and other animal species from neighboring farms should not be allowed into the farm.
9) Feathers, litters and other poultry wastes should be deposited far away from the farmyard. They should be burnt or buried with lime so that they will not be exhumed by scavengers.
10) Management of mixed species of birds should not be practiced. Free-range, wild, exotic and pet birds must be separated from poultry flocks.
11) Visitors to the farms should be limited. When they come, they should be provided with clean and disposable protective clothing. They should not have access to the poultry pens. Poultry houses must not serve as points of sale of birds and birds' products such as eggs.

Basic Biosecurity Measures in Free Range/Scavenging Flocks Systems

Although institution of effective biosecurity measures under the free range/scavenging birds systems might be difficult, keepers must ensure adequate biocontainment principles during disease management.

1) Drugs should not be bought over-the-counter while the attention of veterinary professionals should be sought.
2) Community-led initiatives of movement control can be employed in free range management. This because an individual flock owner cannot do it alone in a village setting with many flocks owners.
3) Contact between free range flocks and migratory birds should be limited.
4) The use of disposable cages should be used for transporting birds to the live bird markets for sale. These cages should be burnt after use.
5) Visits to the live bird markets should be reduced while rest days can be introduced as part of biosecurity measures against HPAI.
6) Interspecies mixing of birds should be highly discouraged both at farm and market levels.
7) Veterinarians should be called upon the advent of unusual diseases.

Early Warning Systems

In some situations, the biosecurity defense line can be breached and this can led to avian influenza outbreaks if adequate surveillance and early warning pointers are not put in place. Early warning systems are control tools for managing the virus outbreaks. They are of utmost importance in the control or suppression of the HPAI H5N1. Early warning systems are developed with the objective of dealing with a disease outbreak in its early stages before it escalates or becomes widespread. Early warning systems rapidly detect the introduction or abrupt rise in incidence of any livestock disease which has the potential to develop epidemic proportions and/or cause serious socioeconomic consequences or public health concerns [41].

In response to the spread of HPAI H5N1, the joint action by the Food and Agriculture Organization (FAO), World Organization for Animal Health (OIE) and World Health Organization (WHO) in 2005 developed integrated early warning system (Global Livestock Early Warning and Response System to Major Transboundary Diseases - GLEWS) that has the potential to thoroughly track the spread of HPAI H5N1 especially in wild birds. FAO, collected, recorded and analyzed data on AI through its Emergency Prevention System for Transboundary Animal and Plant Pests and Diseases program (EMPRES) and the Global Animal Health Information System (EMPRES-i), both in wild bird populations and domestic poultry [41]. Partners and member countries involved receive timely and accurate situation updates on HPAI risk.

Various disease informational materials have hitherto been generated through this action and they include: Disease Tracking List (DTL), ECTAD HPAI Situation Update, Global Information System (GIS) application and the Exploratory Spatial Data Analysis (ESDA).

The information leads to better understanding of the underlying epidemiological and ecological factors responsible for emergence and spread of the disease [41]. However, the use of early warning and early reaction tools is limited in developing countries especially in Africa thereby undermining the effectiveness of these tools in this region. Local and national surveillance programmes do not exist or are limited owing to mismanagement, misappropriation and disorganized activities of all stakeholders involved. To ensure that stakeholders in the poultry industry in developing countries have access to information and risk-assessment outcomes, concerted local, national and internal aids are necessary to achieve the goal of preventing and controlling of HPAI virus in birds. There is need for veterinary capacity development to effectively control virus while also efficient Technical Collaborative efforts are necessary and to be established among various national governmental, non-governmental and international organizations.

CONCLUSION

Areas that have not been affected by an HPAI outbreak or those that have undergone culling, disinfection and even vaccination should improve their biosecurity. Improved biosecurity at whatever level is cost-effective in comparison to the losses from disease, depopulation and further anguish, be it at the village level or commercial farm. The most difficult environment in which to improve biosecurity and disease prevention is likely to be at village level, where poultry and other animals are allowed to move without any restrictions and there are no costs to flock care (feeding), but their losses due to disease or scavenging animals (dogs, cats, wildlife) are high. Under these circumstances, the role of rural developing agencies can be beneficial in promoting the advantages of keeping those animals in a fenced enclosure where environmental stresses are minimized, theft less likely, birds are safer from scavenging animals, and the loss of valued flocks through being run over by motorcycles and vehicles is eliminated. Good biosecurity levels on the farms and in the flocks will ultimately lead to lower costs in the production cycle, and flock welfare will be enhanced. Biosecurity on small-scale poultry farms should emphasize the creation of physical barriers against infection, but because the keepers of free-range flocks cannot act alone, community-led initiatives are necessary. The review findings are plausible as birds from free-range flocks have more opportunities of contact with wild birds that serve as reservoirs of low-pathogenic avian influenza strains than the commercial poultry, thus providing them with constant challenge of flock immunity. The development of efficient and effective biosecurity measures against avian influenza on commercial farms requires adequate placements of barriers to provide segregation, cleaning and disinfection, while concerted community established sanitary measures are needed for free-range poultry flocks in the developing economies. Good biosecurity levels on the farms and in the flocks ultimately lower costs in the production cycle, and flock welfare is always enhanced.

REFERENCES

[1] Normile, D. (2005). Pandemic sceptics warn against crying wolf. *Science*. 310: 1112-1113.

[2] Joannis, T. Lombin, L. H. De Benedictis, P. Catoli, G. and Capua, I. (2006). Confirmation of H5N1 avian influenza in Africa. *Veterinary Journal*. 59: 148–152.

[3] Centre for Infectious Diseases Research and Policy (CIDRAP). (2012). Avian Influenza (Bird Flu): *Agricultural and Wildlife Considerations*. Available at: http://www.cidrap.umnedu/cidrap/. (accessed August 16, 2012).

[4] Kumar, R. Partho Halder, P. and Poddar, R. (2006). Adaptive molecular evolution of virulence genes of avian influenza – A virus subtype H5N1: An analysis of host radiation. *Bioinformation*. 1(8): 321-326.

[5] Fasina, F.O. Bisschop, S.P.R. Ibironke, A.A. and Meseko, C.A. (2009). Avian Influenza Risk Perception among Poultry Workers, Nigeria. *Emerging Infectious Diseases*. 15(4): 616–617.

[6] Breiman, R.F. Nasidi, A. Katz, M.A. Njenga, M.K. and Vertefeuille, J. (2007). Preparedness for Highly Pathogenic Avian Influenza Pandemic in Africa. *Emerging Infectious Diseases*. 13 (10): 1453-1458.

[7] Chang, S-C. Cheng, Y-Y. and Shih, S-R. (2006). Avian Influenza Virus: The Threat of A Pandemic. *Chang Gung Medical Journal*. 29:130-134.

[8] Oxford, J.S. (2000). Influenza A pandemics of the 20th century with special reference to 1918: virology, pathology and epidemiology. *Review of Medical Virology*. 10:119-133.

[9] Hancock, J. and Cho, G. (2008). Assessment of likely impacts of avian influenza on rural poverty reduction in Asia: Responses, impacts and recommendations for IFAD strategy. *International Fund for Agricultural Development* (IFAD) Duscussion paper. 6.

[10] Pan-African Control of Epizootics (PACE). (2006). HPAI in Nigeria: the standard operating procedures, Abuja. *Animal Watch Magazine*. 3: 10–11.

[11] Ugwu, D. A. (2007). Economic impact of avian bird flu on the poultry industry in Nigeria. *Pakistan Journal of Social Science*. 14: 518–524.

[12] Fasina, F.O. Ifende, V.I. and Ajibade, A.A. (2010). Avian influenza A (H5N1) in humans: lessons from Egypt. *European Surveillance*. 15(4): pii=19473. http://www.eurosurveillance.org/ViewArticle.aspx?ArticleId =19473. (Accessed August 16, 2012).

[13] Ibrahim, H. I. Iliyasu, H. Ibrahim, Y. and Siangbe, N.D. (2010). Avian influenza and employment decisions of poultry farmers in the Federal Capital Territory of Nigeria. *Journal of Agricultural Sciences*. 2: 321–324.

[14] Alhaji, N. B. and Odetokun, I. A. (2011). Assessment of Biosecurity Measures Against Highly Pathogenic Avian Influenza Risks in Small-Scale Commercial Farms and Free-Range Poultry Flocks in the Northcentral Nigeria. *Transboundary and Emerging Diseases*. 58: 157–161.

[15] Cattoli, G. Monne, I. Fusaro, A. Joannis, T.M. Lombin, L.H. Aly, M.M. Arafa, A.S. Sturm-Ramirez, K.M. Couacy-Hymann, E. Awuni, J.A. Batawui, K.B. Awoume, K.A. Aplogan, G.L. Sow, A. Ngangnou, A.C. El Nasri Hamza, I.M. Gamatie, D. Dauphin, G. Domenech, J.M. and Capua, I. (2009). Highly Pathogenic Avian Influenza Virus Subtype H5N1 in Africa: *A Comprehensive Phylogenetic Analysis and Molecular Characterization of Isolates*. PLoS ONE 4(3): e4842. doi:10.1371 /journal.pone.0004842.

[16] Hogerwerf, L. Wallace, R.G. Ottaviani, D. Slingenbergh, J. Prosser, D. Bergmann, L. and Gilbert, M. (2010). Persistence of Highly Pathogenic Avian Influenza H5N1 Virus Defined by Agro-Ecological Niche. *Ecohealth*. 7(2): 213–225.

[17] Ducatez, M.F. Olinger, C.M. Owoade, A.A. Tarnagda, Z. Tahita, M.C. Sow, A. De Landtsheer, S. Ammerlaan, W. Ouedraogo, J.B. Osterhaus, A.D.M.E. Fouchier, R. A. M. and Muller, C.P. (2007). Molecular and antigenic evolution and geographical spread of H5N1 highly pathogenic

avian influenza viruses in western Africa. *Journal of General Virology*. 88: 2297–2306.

[18] Dodman, T. (2006). Waterbird family estimates in Africa. Waterbird population estimates. 4th edition. Wageningen (the Netherlands): *Wetlands International*.

[19] Gaidet, N. Dodman, T. Caron, A. Balança, G. Desvaux, S. Goutard, F. Cattoli, G. Lamarque, F. Hagemeijer, W. and Monicat, F. (2007). Avian Influenza Viruses in Water Birds, Africa. *Emerging Infectious Diseases*. 13(4): 626-629.

[20] Musa, O. I. Salaudeen, A.G. Akanbi, I.I. and Bolarinwa, O.A. (2009). Risk factors, threats and prevention of highly pathogenic avian influenza (HPAI) in African countries. *African Journal of Clinical and Experimental Microbiology*. 10: 99–116.

[21] Musa, O.I. Aderibigbe, S.A. Salaudeen, G.A. Oluwole, F.A. and Samuel, S.O. (2010). Community awareness of bird flu and the practice of backyard poultry in a North-Central State of Nigeria. *Journal of Preventive Medicine and Hygiene*. 51: 146-151.

[22] Otte, J. Pfeiffer, D. Tiensin, T. Price, L. and Silbergeld, E. (2007). Highly pathogenic avian influenza risk, biosecurity and smallholder adversity. *Livestock Research for Rural Development. 19 (7): 102.* http://www.lrrd.org/lrrd19/7/otte19102.htm. *(Accessed* July 20, 2012).

[23] Grabkowsky, B. (2009). *Strategies for prevention, monitoring and control of avian influenza at farm level*. Available at: http://www.thepoultrysite.com/articles/1421/. (Accessed June 13, 2009).

[24] Gerba, C. and Smith, J. E. (2005). Sources of pathogenic micro-organisms and their fate during land application of wastes. *Journal of Environmental Quality*. 34: 42-48.

[25] Jones, T. Donnelly, C. and Stamp Dawkins, M. (2005). Environmental and management factors affecting the welfare of chickens on commercial farms in the United Kingdom and Denmark stocked at five densities. *Poultry Science*. 84: 1155-1165.

[26] Gilbert, M. Chaitaweesub, P. Parakamawongsa, T. Premashthira, S. Tiensin, T. Kalpravidh, W. Wagner, H. and Slingenbergh, J. (2006). Free-grazing ducks and highly pathogenic avian influenza, Thailand. *Emerging Infectious Diseases*. 12: 227-234.

[27] Lebarbenchon, C. Feare, C.J. Renaud, F. Thomas, F. and Gauthier-Clerc, M. (2010). Persistence of Highly Pathogenic Avian Influenza Viruses in Natural Ecosystems. *Emerging Infectious Diseases*. 16 (7): 1057-1062.

[28] Marangon, S. Capua, I. Rossi, E.J. Ferré, N. Dalla Pozza, M. Bonfanti, L. and Mannelli, A. (2005). The control of avian influenza in areas at risk: the Italian experience 1997-2003. In: Avian Influenza: *Prevention and Control* (Vol. 8). Schrijver, Remco S.; Koch, G. (Eds.), IX, 152 p.
[29] Capua, I. and Marangon, S. (2006). Control of Avian Influenza in Poultry. *Emerging Infectious Diseases*. 12 (9): 1319-1324.
[30] De Benedictis, P. Beato, M.S. and Capua, I. (2007). Inactivation of Avian Influenza Viruses by Chemical Agents and Physical Conditions: A Review. *Zoonoses and Public Health*. 54: 51–68.
[31] Charisis, N. (2008). Avian influenza biosecurity: a key for animal and human protection. *Veterinaria Italiana*. 44 (4): 657-669.
[32] Food and Agriculture Organization (FAO). (2008). Biosecurity for Highly Pathogenic Avian Influenza: *Issues and options*. FAO Animal Production and Health Paper No. 165. http://www.fao.org/docrep/011/i0359e/i0359e00.htm. (Accessed August 16, 2012).
[33] Xiang, N. Shi, Y. Wu, J. Zhang, S. Ye, M. Peng, Z. Zhou, L. Zhou, H. Liao, Q. Huai, Y. Li, L. Yu, Z. Cheng, X. Su, W. Wu, X. Ma, H. Lu, J. McFarland, J. and Yu, H. (2010). Knowledge, attitudes and practices (KAP) relating to avian influenza in urban and rural areas of China. *BMC Infectious Diseases*. 10:34.
[34] Federal Government of Nigeria (FGN). (2007). Avian Influenza Control and Human Pandemic Preparedness and Response Project National Baseline Survey. Final Report. *EnvironQuest Integrated Environmental Solutions*. Available at. http://www.aicpnigeria.org/documents/AICP%20Baseline%20Survey.pdf (Accessed 26/8/2012).
[35] Maris, P. (1995). *Mode of action of disinfectants*. Revue Scientifique et Technique.14: 47–55.
[36] Wanaratana, S. Tantilertcharoen, R. Sasipreeyaian, J. and Pakpinyo, S. (2010). The inactivation of avian influenza virus subtype H5N1 isolated from chickens in Thailand by chemical and physical treatments. *Veterinary Microbiology* 140: 43-48.
[37] World Health Organization (WHO). (2006). Collecting, preserving and shipping specimens for the diagnosis of avian influenza A (H5N1) virus infection: Guide for field operations. *Epidemic and pandemic alert and response*. WHO/CDS/EPR/ARO/2006.1. http://www.who.int/csr/resources/publications/surveillance/CDS_EPR_ARO_2006_1.pdf (Accessed 26/08/2012).

[38] Vong, S. Ly, S. Mardy S. Holl, D. and Buchy, P. (2008). Environmental contamination during influenza A virus (H5N1) outbreaks, Cambodia. *Emerging Infectious Diseases*. 14:1303–1305.

[39] Chaichoune, K. Wiriyarat, W. Thitithanyanont, A. Phonarknguen, R. Sariya, L. Suwanpakdee, S. Noimor, T. Chatsurachai, S. Suriyaphol, P. Ungchusak, K. Ratanakorn, P. Webster, R.G. Thompson, M. Auewarakul, P. and Puthavathana, P. (2009). Indigenous sources of 2007-2008 H5N1 avian influenza outbreaks in Thailand. *Journal of General Virology*. 90(1): 216-22.

[40] Food and Agriculture Organization (FAO). (2004). Recommendations on the prevention, control, and eradication of highly pathogenic avian influenza (HPAI) in Asia. F*ood and Agriculture Organization of the United Nations*, Rome, Italy. http://web.oie.int/eng/AVIAN_INFLUENZA/FAO%20recommendations%20on%20HPAI.pdf (Accessed August 16, 2012).

[41] Martin, V. von Dobschuetz, S. Lemenach, A. N. Schoustra, W. and DeSimone, L. (2007). Early Warning, Database, and Information Systems for Avian Influenza Surveillance. *Journal of Wildlife Diseases*. 43(3): S71–S76.

In: Avian Influenza ISBN: 978-1-62417-415-5
Editors: K. M. Taylor and B. O'Connor

Chapter 3

OUTBREAK CONTROL AND VIRAL EVOLUTION OF THE HIGHLY PATHOGENIC H5N1 AVIAN INFLUENZA IN THAILAND

Witthawat Wiriyarat, Kridsada Chaichoune, Parntep Ratanakorn and Prasert Auewarakul

Monitoring and Surveillance Center for Zoonotic Diseases in Wildlife and Exotic Animals (MoZWE) and Center for Emerging and Neglected Infectious Diseases (CENID), Mahidol University, Nakhon Pathom, Thailand

ABSTRACT

Thailand is known for its success in controlling the highly pathogenic H5N1 avian influenza epidemic. Despite the explosive outbreak in 2003-2004 similar to other countries in the East and Southeast Asian region, the epidemic was bought down under control in 2006 with the elimination of infectious sources by "stamping out", strengthened biosecurity measures, and periodic active surveillance as the main control strategies. The initial epidemic in 2003-2005 involved mainly medium to large scale farming, resulting in massive economic loss. After 2006, sporadic cases occurred seasonally in backyard poultry in certain repeated outbreak areas involving limited number of poultry. The last animal outbreak was reported in 2008, and the last indigenous human case was detected in 2006. The reduction of viral population size was also evidenced by the reduced viral sequence diversity after 2006. The viral sequences showed little changes without evidences of positive selection during this low level endemic period and no known human-adapted mutations were observed. Similarity of viral sequences among outbreak seasons indicated that the virus was maintained in a local reservoir between outbreak seasons. Virus of similar lineage was occasionally isolated from local wild birds and migratory birds. Although some of these birds migrate in a route covering Southeast Asia to the epidemic hot spots in Central Asia, the similarity of viral sequences in these birds to the local virus suggested that the birds acquired the virus locally rather than carrying new viruses into the country. The small reservoir size in a limited area suggested that the virus can be eradicated from the country. While the current situation in the country is well under control, new kindle from undetected local reservoirs and import of new viral strains through human or wildlife activities are still a threat.

INTRODUCTION

Thailand was severely affected by the initial H5N1 highly pathogenic avian influenza (HPAI) outbreak of Southeast Asia. The virus spread to many countries and established endemicity. While many countries with large scale outbreak are able to bring the outbreak under partial control, some countries are still having active outbreak. However, eradication is not considered to be achievable and low level endemicity with sporadic outbreaks is believed to a norm in these countries [1]. In Thailand, the outbreak gradually declined in every outbreak season. Outbreak has not been detected since 2007, and only a small number of viruses were detected in active surveillance programs. While it is still to see whether eradication will be achieved, it is clear that the outbreak in Thailand is now well under control. Learning from this success may be helpful for the control of outbreaks in other countries.

THE EPIDEMIC

After the successful control of the initial outbreak of H5N1 highly pathogenic avian influenza virus in 1997 in Hong Kong by depopulating all the poultry on the island, the virus was only sporadically detected in Southern China until 2003 [2]. In autumn of 2003, outbreaks of H5N1 HPAI were reported from Korea, Japan and then Vietnam [3]. In October 2003, poultry die-off was reported from many provinces in Thailand. The causative organism was initially reported to be *Pasteurella multocida* (avian cholera). Despite the attempt to control the outbreak by destroying affected flocks, the outbreak continued to expand throughout the winter of 2003 to all the regions of the country. It was not until the first human case was diagnosed in January 2004 that the causative agent of the poultry outbreaks was confirmed to be H5N1 HPAI [4]. The first wave of outbreaks subsided in April 2004, when summer started, and disappeared in May. In this first outbreak season, 190 outbreaks were reported from 89 districts of 42 provinces scattering all over the country [5]. About 60 millions poultry were destroyed in this first episode. The decline of the epidemic in summer was probably because the high temperature and low humidity in summer was not suitable for the viral transmission. Before the disappearance of the outbreak in summer, the virus had probably already seeded itself in many areas throughout the country. After a few quiet months, the rainy season came and outbreaks started again in July 2004. This second wave of epidemic was explosive with reports of 1539 outbreaks in 264 districts of 51 provinces (of 76 provinces of Thailand). The outbreaks involved all types of poultry, especially medium and large scale farming. Although outbreaks were reported from all regions of the country, the most heavily affected areas were in the Central and Lower Northern regions [5]. Free-grazing ducks, which are commonly raised in paddy fields, were also affected [6]. The epidemic had severe economic, social and political impacts on the country. Before 2004, Thailand was a major exporter of poultry with over 1.5 billion US$ export per annum. This figure was about 1.4% of total export and 0.8% of GDP. With the ongoing epidemic in the country, export of poultry meat dramatically decreased and only cooked poultry products were exported. Domestic consumption of poultry and eggs also reduced dramatically. These severely affected the poultry economic sector of the country. The lesson that should be learned from this explosive epidemic in 2004 is that by not responding drastically and effectively to the initial outbreaks in 2003, the virus was allowed to spread extensively throughout the country leading to the large scale outbreaks that severely affected the economy of the country for many years. In comparison, Korea and Japan, which experienced H5N1 HAPAI outbreaks in 2003, responded swiftly to the outbreaks and had the outbreaks controlled or eradicated with only limited impact.

After the explosive outbreaks in 2004, the epidemic strictly followed a seasonal epidemic curve, starting in rainy season with a peak in late rainy season/early winter and subsiding as the weather warmed up in summer [7, 8]

(Thailand has three seasons: rainy season in June – September, winter in October – January, and summer in February – May). With each passing outbreak season, the epidemic became smaller both in number of affected animals and localization of outbreaks. The Central area with river basins was the area with repeated outbreaks [9]. Limited outbreaks by a different strain of virus also occurred in the Northeastern region bordering Laos [10]. After 2006, only limited sporadic outbreaks involving small number of animals, mostly backyard poultry, were detected. And, no outbreak was reported since 2008.

THE TRANSMISSION DYNAMICS

In the early phase of epidemic in 2003 - 2004, industrial farming was heavily affected. Because of the high density farming system, the virus spread though a flock very quickly resulting in massive death within a few days. Cumulative mortality in a flock can progress rapidly from 2% within one day of the appearance of clinical signs to 100% within 6 days [11]. The basic reproductive number (R_0) of this intra-flock transmission was estimated to be not very high (2.26 – 2.64) [11]. Nevertheless, the transmission can be very fast because of the short generation time. The upper bound of the R_0 was estimated to be 5 [11]. This number has an implication on the preventive strategy since the basic reproductive number dictates the threshold of herd immunity required for protection of the herd ($1-1/R_0$). The level of herd immunity or the vaccine coverage in the case of $R_0 = 5$ is 80%. Interesting interaction between intensive farming and backyard poultry in the viral transmission and outbreak perpetuation was observed in the epidemic of 2004. While high-density farming served as the source of high contagiousness, farm to farm transmission was not sufficient for the transmission chain and backyard poultry might play a role to sustain the transmission chain [12]. The lower population density and contact rate in backyard poultry and the ability of ducks to shred the virus over an extended period protracted the transmission chain and enabled the maintenance of the virus within or among interacting populations [13-15]. Spatio-temporal analyses of outbreaks suggested that transmission among farms was highly localized and involved human activities [16-19]. More than 90% of cases had a previous case within a 10 km range and a 21 day period of time. The maximum distance of transmission between farms was estimated to be lower than 60 kilometers [18]. Long-distance poultry transportation might play a crucial role in broadening the outbreak zone. In addition to movement of poultry to and from farms for production and marketing, movement of free-grazing ducks by trucks to new paddy fields for feeding and movement of fighting cocks between fighting tournaments contributed to the spread in the early phase of epidemic. Several risk analyses showed consistently that density of free-grazing ducks and rice paddy fields were associated with outbreaks [19-21]. Other anthropogenic factors, such as densely populated areas, short distances to a highway junction, and short distances to large cities were associated with HPAI outbreaks [17]. In addition, bringing live chickens from another backyard farm was associated with an increased risk of HPAI in backyard flocks [22]. These together suggest a complex interaction among the components of outbreak leading to successful spreading of HPAI in a large scale epidemic (Figure 1a). The role of free-living birds in the epidemic is not yet clear. Although HPAI detection rate in free-living birds was higher in outbreak areas when the outbreaks were active, it is not known whether this represented only a spill-over from poultry outbreaks into bird populations or those infected birds played a role of carrying virus between farms or backyard flocks. Infection rate in free-living birds was mostly low ranging from 0.5% to 2.7% [23]. An exception was the outbreaks in open-billed stork colonies in 2004 and 2005. This species lives in high density colonies and is highly susceptible to H5N1 HPAI infection with high mortality.

The intra-flock transmission in open-billed storks probably resembled the transmission in high-density farms owing to the high-density nesting behavior of this species. Similar to the situation in high-density farming, rapid and effective intra-flock transmission made intra-flock sustained transmission chain unlikely and most outbreaks resulted in depopulation to the point that the transmission chain could be no longer sustained due to the reduction of population density and contact rate.

In accordance with this hypothesis, analysis of viral sequences from open-billed stork colonies suggested new introduction of virus into the colonies in each outbreak season, and no evidence of sustaining the virus in the colonies for longer than an outbreak season (Chaichoune, unpublished data).

In contrast to the explosive outbreaks of 2004, the epidemic seasons of 2006 and the subsequent years mainly involved backyard poultry and were much less in intensity [24]. Strengthened biosecurity was likely the major factor preventing transmission into industrial farming sector, whereas intensive surveillance and elimination of infectious sources limited the viral spread among backyard flocks.

Prohibition of poultry movement across regions also probably played an important role to limit the extent of viral spread, especially from free-grazing duck flocks and fighting cocks [6]. These factors together reduced the epidemic to a low endemicity level (Figure 1b).

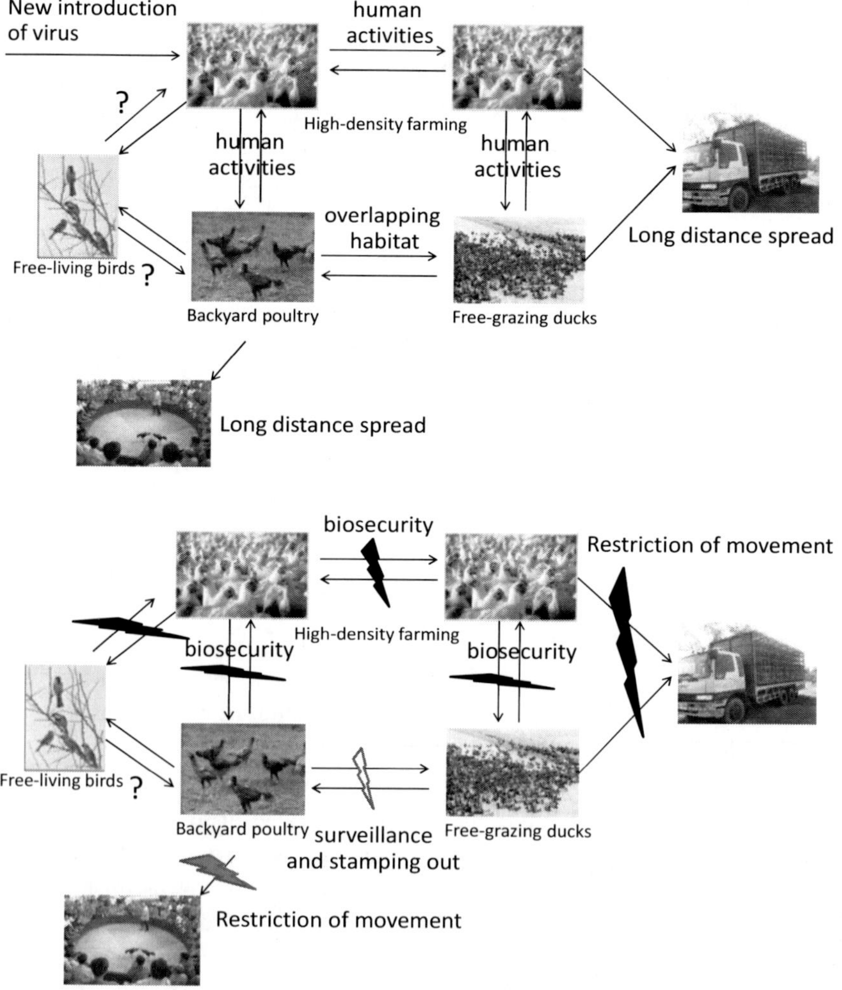

Figure 1. Successful spreading of HPAI in a large scale epidemic in 2003-2005 with local transmission among industrial farms, backyard poultry, free-grazing ducks, free-living birds; and long-range transmission by poultry trade and movement of fighting cocks (a). After 2006, the epidemic was substantial reduced to a low endemic level by the control measures, which include strengthened biosecurity in the industrial farming sector, surveillance, and restriction of poultry movement (b).

THE CONTROL MEASURES

Different countries utilized different strategies in combating the H5N1 HPAI epidemic. The most obvious difference is the use of vaccine. While many countries use vaccine either aiming at extensive vaccine coverage or ring vaccination to prevent spread from detected outbreaks, Thailand prohibits HPAI vaccine. While the main reason for this decision was probably influenced by the policy of major importing countries not to import poultry products from any country that uses HPAI vaccine, scientific reason for the prohibition of HPAI vaccine was the fear for inapparent infection in partially immuned animals, which would complicate the surveillance and effectiveness of the infectious source elimination. Although HPAI vaccine is officially prohibited, whether and how extensive illegal vaccine usage was practiced is not known. It is likely that smuggled vaccine was used in some layer hen farms and fighting cocks. Without the help of vaccine, the national outbreak control strategy relied mainly on 1) active and passive surveillance, 2) stamping out infected flocks, and 3) Prohibition of poultry movement.

Active and Passive Surveillance

Since 2004, Thailand has spent a lot of effort in strengthening the avian influenza surveillance system. The surveillance system was carried out based on clinical observation and laboratory diagnosis, which were mainly responsible by the Department of Livestock Development (DLD), Ministry of Agriculture and Cooperatives [25]. In addition, a surveillance collaborative network, comprising of Ministry of Agriculture and Cooperatives, Ministry of Public Health, Ministry of Natural Resource and Environment, Ministry of Interior as well as Universities, has been established to ensure effective cooperation and sufficient resources. Different surveillance strategies were implemented during non-epidemic and epidemic phase. During non-epidemic phase, continuous passive surveillance using clinical criteria for unusual poultry death and a periodic active surveillance system called "X-ray campaign" were the main mechanisms. For clinical HPAI surveillance, the criteria of suspected HPAI cases according to the DLD's definition are as follows: 1) death rate at least 1% within 2 days for poultry in farms or the water and feed consumption rates decreased by 20% within 1 day, or 2) death rate at least 5% within 2 days for backyard poultry, and 3) clinical signs compatible with HPAI, which include respiratory distress, depress, inappetite, swelling of face and tearing, seizure, ruffled feathers, reduction of eggs, diarrhea, petechial hemorrhages on shanks, cyanosis of wattles and combs and sudden death. Once any unusual illness and death of poultry that met the clinical HPAI case definition was found, village health volunteers (VHV) or local DLD staffs would notify DLD local officers who would visit the site and approve culling or a "stamping-out" of the suspected poultry immediately without a laboratory result and animal owners would receive a compensation at 75% of the market value. The aim of this activity is to control HPAI spreading as swiftly as possible without a delay by laboratory investigation. However, samples from suspected cases were collected for laboratory testing. And, if H5N1 HPAI was detected, an intensive survey and outbreak control measures would be implemented. Additional samples would be collected from poultry in every farm or household in the area of 5 kilometer (km) radius surrounding the beginning outbreak area. Thereafter, if an additional positive case was found, a new 5 km-radius area would be established around the new case. VHVs are villagers who have been elected and trained in primary health care. VHUs are instrumental in implementing primary healthcare measures and communicating with villagers on healthcare issues. VHV is an integral part of the Thai healthcare system for over 30 years. There are currently more than 800,000 VHVs in the country, and one VHU is responsible for 8 – 15 household in the rural areas. The strength of the VHV system contributed significantly to the success of the clinical surveillance. In addition, a passive surveillance was carried out by monitoring laboratory testing results from all veterinary laboratories throughout the country. Those laboratories tested poultry samples from pre-slaughtering, pre-movement, and farm health monitoring programs.

In addition to the routine surveillance program, an active intensive surveillance known as "X-ray campaign" was carried out at least twice a year. During the campaign, VHVs and village livestock volunteers visited every household in villages for HPAI clinical active surveillance to identify sick or dead birds. Daily reports of unusual sick or dead animals including humans or negative reports were submitted to HPAI reporting system of the DLD. In addition, active laboratory surveillance was conducted by the National Institute of Animal Health (NIAH) and Regional Veterinary Diagnosis and Research Centers. Cloacal swabs were systematically sampled from poultry throughout the country, especially in HPAI repeated outbreak areas, and tested for H5N1 HPAI. For example, during the first X-ray campaign in October 2004, a total of 150,648 samples were collected, 724 (0.48%) samples from 457 sub-districts, 184 districts, 44 provinces were found to be positive for

H5N1 HPAI. The second X-ray campaign was performed on 1-28 February 2005. A total of 66,588 samples were tested, 72 (0.1%) samples from 37 sub-districts, 22 districts, 10 provinces were found to be positive. The third X-ray activity was performed on 1-31 July 2005, a total of 84,954 samples were collected and 20 (0.023%) samples from 17 sub-districts, 7 districts, 3 provinces were found to be positive [5]. The campaign has been continued regularly twice a year. The timing of the campaigns is usually set at the beginning and the end of each outbreak season. The timing of the campaign in January – February is not only intended for the end of the outbreak season but also to the timing of the Chinese New Year, when there are a lot out poultry movement for market demand.

During epidemic phase, controlling the spreading of outbreaks is the top priority. At the outbreak site and 5 km-radius surrounding area, intensive laboratory surveillance was implemented by collecting samples from farms, household flocks, and wild birds in the area for laboratory investigation. All poultry at the outbreak site were destroyed, and poultry movement was prohibited within 10 km radius surrounding outbreak area. Disinfection of the outbreak area was also carried out by chemical spray. In addition, active clinical surveillance was performed by VHVs, local DLD staff and all villagers within 10 km radius surrounding the outbreak area. The role of VHV is one of the key success factors in HPAI outbreak control in Thailand. VHVs played very active roles not only in the clinical surveillance and early warning, but also in enforcing poultry quarantine, assisting sample collection and promoting awareness.

Stamping out

As HPAI vaccination is prohibited in Thailand, ring vaccination cannot be implemented and poultry depopulation in and surrounding outbreak areas is the only direct control measure. In combination with compensation at 75% of local market price, stamping out is well accepted by poultry owners. At the beginning of HPAI outbreak in Thailand, poultry depopulation was carried out for all types of poultry (broiler chickens, layer chickens, backyard chickens, ducks, quails, turkeys, ostriches) in an area of 5 km radius surrounding outbreak sites. After the initial two months of the epidemic, the scale of the outbreaks was substantially reduced, and the method of poultry stamping out was modified. Only the poultry in the affected premises were depopulated and samples were collected from animals within 5 km-radius area for laboratory testing. Poultry movement was prohibited and active HPAI clinical survey was performed in the 10 km-radius area. Animal culling was practiced by well-trained staff of DLD and Thai Armed Forces by using CO_2. The total number of animal destroyed in the first three big wave of HPAI outbreak during January, 2004 to November, 2005 is 64,460,504. These were sum of 60,811,081 animals in the first outbreak (winter 2004), 3,232,277 animals in second wave of outbreak (rainy season 2005) and 417,146 animals in the third wave (winter 2005).

Prohibition of Poultry Movement

Transportation of poultry and poultry products was identified as a major route to disseminate H5N1 HPAI [17]. Thus, poultry movement prohibition is an importance measure for the outbreak control in Thailand. The government set up five poultry movement restriction zones according to the geographic regions of Thailand (North, Central, North-East, East, and South). During outbreaks, movement of poultry out of 10 km radius surrounding the outbreak sites but within the movement restriction zones was prohibited for at least 30 days, whereas transportation to other zones was not allowed for at least 60 days. The transportation can be resumed after the HPAI was completely cleared from the area and animal owners need permission from authorized DLD officers before moving their poultry. However, the zoning practices is only practical for small scale poultry producers who sell their product locally but not for the industrial farming sector. Poultry export is an important economic activity of Thailand. In 2003, before the HPAI epidemic, Thailand exported 545,987 tons of poultry products with a value of 48,418 million Baht or US$1,618.8 million. Fortunately, World Organization for Animal Health (OIE) introduced the “compartmentalization” concept in 2005. OIE recognized that OIE member countries may face difficulties in establishing and maintaining a diseases free status for the whole country, especially in the case of diseases that can easily cross international boundaries (OIE Terrestrial Animal Health Code Chapter 4.4). The concept of compartmentalization is that domestic livestock can be effectively raised and isolated from other kinds of mammals, birds and wildlife, and the animals or products derived from livestock within these isolated compartments can be safely traded [26]. The concept of compartmentalization allowed poultry producers to create compartments that contain subpopulations of disease-free animals, which may be in different locations but are maintained under a common good biosecurity management system [27]. OIE defines a 'compartment' as "an animal subpopulation contained in one or more establishments under a common biosecurity management system with a distinct health status with respect to a specific disease or diseases for which required surveillance, control and biosecurity measures have been applied for the purpose of international trade" [28]. To ensure that the subpopulation in the compartment complies with the defined health status, surveillance programs must be implemented. Many different combinations of testing and surveillance may be applied to gain the necessary confidence with regard to freedom from the disease. In order to comply with this concept, commercial poultry producers must have effective biosecurity and surveillance programs and receive certifications from DLD for a Notifiable AI-Free Compartment and for maintenance of the Notifiable AI-Free Compartment status.

VIRUS IN VARIOUS SPECIES

H5N1 HPAI has a very wide host range. Numerous species have been reported to be susceptible to H5N1 HPAI. While feline species including domestic cats (*Felis sylvestris catus*), leopard (*Panthera pardus*), and tiger (*Panthera tigris tigris*) are highly susceptible to the infection and severe disease [29, 30], domestic pigs (*Sus domestica*) are resistant to the infection and do not transmit the virus efficiently [31]. Among avian species, variable degrees of susceptibility were also observed, for example feral pigeons (*Columba livia*) are more resistant and require highly viral dose for the infection, whereas chicken (*Gallus gallus*), Japanese quails (*Coturnix coturnix japonica*), sparrows *(Passer domesticus)* and open-billed storks (*Anasthomus oscitans*) are highly susceptible [32-36].

Except for the outbreak in open-billed stork colonies, outbreak in other free-living bird species has not been observed in Thailand. Active surveillance data in free-living bird species showed a low level of infection rate in various species [23]. Birds species commonly found to be infected were rock pigeon (*Columba livia*), tree sparrow (*Passer montanus*), common myna (*Acridotheres tristis*), Asian pied starling (*Sturnus contra*), common koel (*Eudynamys scolopacea*), white-vented myna (*Acridotheres grandis*), scaly-breasted munia (*Lonchura punctulata*), lesser whistling-duck (*Dendrocygna javanica*). These are common species living in proximity to humans and poultry and probably contracted the virus from poultry. Viral sequences from these free-living birds were phylogenetically separable from poultry viruses

[37]. Some association between high viral detection rate in birds and poultry outbreaks was observed suggesting the role of these birds in transmitting the virus. In addition, some rodents may get infected by feeding on chicken carcasses and carry the virus from flock to flock.

Long-range migratory birds were shown to be the viral carrier for the H5N1 HPAI spread from Western China to Europe. Many bird species migrate to Thailand in winter, when the HPAI outbreak season is active, and are at high risk of contracting the infection. Some of these species were studies for the presence of H5N1 HPAI infection. The virus was detected in some brown-headed gulls. The similarity of viral sequences in these birds to the local virus suggested that the birds acquired the virus locally rather than carrying new viruses into the country. Brown-headed gulls were shown by satellite telemetry to migrate from Qinghai lake area in Western China, a H5N1 HPAI hot spot, to Bangladesh and the Gulf of Thailand (Rattanakorn, manuscript in preparation). Whether they can carry a HPAI virus over the distance of the migratory route is not known.

The Viral Evolution

Evolution of H5N1 HPAI is complex and involved both rapid mutation and reassortment of genomic segments among avian influenza strains. Multiple genomic constellations of H5N1 HPAI as defined as "genotype" were described, and the initial explosive outbreak in Southeast Asia was caused by the genotype Z [2]. Mutation and divergence of the viral hemagglutinin (HA) sequences resulted in emergence of ten different clades of viruses. Some clades are further classified into subclades [38, 39]. Although these clades showed some differences in their antigenic property, whether the immune selection pressure contributed to the emergence of the clades is unclear. The virus that caused the initial epidemic in Thailand was clade 1 virus. Some evidences suggested that this virus was originated from Yunnan in Southern China [40]. This virus circulated mainly Thailand, Cambodia, and Vietnam. While the clade 1 virus is still circulating in Cambodia, it gradually disappeared from Thailand and in Vietnam it was replaced by viruses of different clades [41]. How the virus spread from Yunnan to Thailand and Vietnam is unclear. There is no evidence that long-range migratory birds were responsible for this spread. On the other hand, the fact that the initial outbreaks occurred in large-scale farms suggested that inter-country trade and transportation of contaminated products or poultry might be the main route of the spread. In the subsequent years after the initial outbreak season of 2004, the clade 1 virus was confined to a few provinces in upper Central and lower Northern regions in the Yom-Nan river basin [42]. In 2006, another strain of virus caused outbreaks in Northeastern provinces bordering Laos along the Mekong river. This virus belonged to clade 2.3.4 [10]. While the virus continued to circulate in Laos, it has not been detected in Northeast Thailand since 2007.

Because H5N1 HPAI is a new virus, which may have gone through an adaptation to new hosts and transmission environments, analyses of positive selection in the viral genomes may help us to understand the adaptation process. Understanding the viral evolution may give us an insight into the mechanism of viral emergence. Although the H5N1 HPAI can infect and cause disease in humans, it cannot transmit efficiently from human to human. This may be viewed as an incomplete adaptation to human host. If further adaptation occurs, a pandemic strain may be emerged. Viral adaptation and positive selection in the viral genome is therefore of great interest. Evidences of positive selection can be analyzed by dN/dS (non-synonymous changes/ synonymous changes) ratio. A dN/dS ratio of more than 1 indicates positive selection. Analyses of viral sequences from Thailand, Vietnam, and Indonesia in 2003 - 2005 showed evidences of positive selection (dN/dS > 1) in M2 and PB1F2 genes [43]. In contrast, more recent viruses of 2006 - 2010 did not show any positive selection in the M2 gene, but showed a higher degree of positive selection the PB1F2 gene. This high dN/dS in PB1-F2 is difficult to interpret and may be interfered by the overlapping PB1 open reading frame. Although it is uncertain whether the high dN/dS in PB1-F2 of the recent virus group really means a positive selection, it can be inferred that the recent virus group either had an increased positive selection or became less constrained as compared to the early virus group. The difference in the pattern of positive selection in the genome of the early viruses and the more recent viruses suggests a change in the viral evolution from actively adapting to new environments in the early phase toward equilibrium, where the virus is optimal for the existence in the current conditions (Kongchanagul, Acta Virol in press).

Large scale vaccination programs were implemented in some countries. Immunological selective pressure is expected to drive rapid changes in viral immunological characteristics. This was one of the arguments against vaccine usage in Thailand. It is, however, unclear how much this selective pressure affected the viral evolution. A recent study comparing countries that used (Egypt, Indonesia) and did not used HPAI vaccine (Nigeria, Turkey, Thailand) found evidences of stronger positive selection in the viral HA gene in those countries using HPAI vaccine [44].

Phylogenetic analyses of the clade 1 viral sequences from Thailand in 2004 - 2005 showed diverse multiple branches, which did not correlate with host species or geographical areas, except for certain groups of viruses causing large outbreaks in open-billed stork colonies. These diverse multiple branches are characteristic of exponential growth of viral population with weak or no selective pressure. Despite this diversity, the virus did not form distinct subclades. This is in contrast to the clade 2 virus in Indonesia, which started the epidemic at about the same time, but evolved to form multiple subclades [38, 43]. This is probably because outbreaks in Indonesia were less interconnecting and could provide local separation of outbreaks from one another leading to spatial structure of the viral population and emergence of subclades. In contrast to the diversity in the 2005 – 2006 outbreaks, viruses in 2006 and the subsequent years were more homogeneous [42]. The reason for the reduced viral diversity in the later years was because of the reduction in viral population size and a bottle-neck effect. HPAI outbreaks in Thailand have a strong seasonality. During the hot and dry summer months, outbreak completely disappeared and active surveillance usually failed to isolate the virus. It is clear that this inter-outbreak period exert a strong bottle-neck effect on the viral population, and only a small number of virus survived to continue the transmission chain in the subsequent season [42]. Phylogenetic analyses of viral sequences of 2007 – 2008 showed not only that the viral sequences belonged to only a couple of lineages but also that there were reassortments among the lineages [45]. This suggested that these residual viruses were sustained in the same group of hosts, and that eradication may be possible if the carriers of these residual viruses can be identified and eliminated.

Conclusion

Thailand experienced a large scale outbreak of H5N1 HPAI in 2004. The outbreak was brought under control in 2005, and only sporadic cases were detected after 2006. The control measures include compartmentalization of poultry population into geographical regions and production sectors; strengthened biosecurity in industrial farming; and intensive surveillance and infectious source elimination by stamping out. While some other countries that experienced similar outbreak are still struggling to control the outbreak, Thailand has been free from HPAI outbreak since 2008, and the last detectable virus was reported in 2010. In agreement with the epidemiological data, viral sequence analyses indicate that viral population size became very small. Whether this indicates a successful eradication is still to be seen. However, these experiences showed us that bringing a nation-wide HPAI epidemic under control is achievable without implementation of a vaccination program and even eradication may be feasible.

REFERENCES

[1] Brown, I.H., Summary of avian influenza activity in Europe, Asia, and Africa, 2006-2009. Avian Dis, 2010. 54(1 Suppl): p. 187-93.

[2] Li, K.S., et al., Genesis of a highly pathogenic and potentially pandemic H5N1 influenza virus in eastern Asia. *Nature*, 2004. 430(6996): p. 209-13.

[3] Outbreaks of avian influenza A (H5N1) in Asia and interim recommendations for evaluation and reporting of suspected cases--United States, 2004. *MMWR Morb. Mortal Wkly Rep.*, 2004. 53(5): p. 97-100.

[4] Cases of influenza A (H5N1)--Thailand, 2004. *MMWR Morb. Mortal Wkly Rep.*, 2004. 53(5): p. 100-3.

[5] (DLD)., D.o.L.D. Avian Influenza Control Center: daily situation; January 1, 2009. Bangkok: DLD, 2009e. [Cited 2009 Jan 1]. Available from: URL: http://www.dld.go.th/home/ bird_flu/birdflu.html. 2009 July 9, 2012].

[6] Songserm, T., et al., Domestic ducks and H5N1 influenza epidemic, Thailand. *Emerg Infect Dis.*, 2006. 12(4): p. 575-81.

[7] Buranathai, C., et al., Surveillance activities and molecular analysis of H5N1 highly pathogenic avian influenza viruses from Thailand, 2004-2005. *Avian Dis.*, 2007. 51(1 Suppl): p. 194-200.

[8] Tiensin, T., et al., Highly pathogenic avian influenza H5N1, Thailand, 2004. *Emerg Infect Dis.*, 2005. 11(11): p. 1664-72.

[9] Tiensin, T., et al., Geographic and temporal distribution of highly pathogenic avian influenza A virus (H5N1) in Thailand, 2004-2005: an overview. *Avian Dis.,* 2007. 51(1 Suppl): p. 182-8.

[10] Chutinimitkul, S., et al., New strain of influenza A virus (H5N1), Thailand. *Emerg Infect Dis.*, 2007. 13(3): p. 506-7.

[11] Tiensin, T., et al., Transmission of the highly pathogenic avian influenza virus H5N1 within flocks during the 2004 epidemic in Thailand. *J. Infect Dis.,* 2007. 196(11): p. 1679-84.

[12] Walker, P., et al., Outbreaks of H5N1 in poultry in Thailand: the relative role of poultry production types in sustaining transmission and the impact of active surveillance in control. *J. R. Soc. Interface*, 2012. 9(73): p. 1836-45.

[13] Hulse-Post, D.J., et al., Role of domestic ducks in the propagation and biological evolution of highly pathogenic H5N1 influenza viruses in Asia. *Proc. Natl. Acad. Sci. USA,* 2005. 102(30): p. 10682-7.

[14] Kim, J.K., et al., Ducks: the "Trojan horses" of H5N1 influenza. *Influenza Other Respi Viruses*, 2009. 3(4): p. 121-8.

[15] Sturm-Ramirez, K.M., et al., Are ducks contributing to the endemicity of highly pathogenic H5N1 influenza virus in Asia? *J. Virol.*, 2005. 79(17): p. 11269-79.

[16] Marquetoux, N., et al., Estimating spatial and temporal variations of the reproduction number for highly pathogenic avian influenza H5N1 epidemic in Thailand. *Prev. Vet. Med.*, 2012.

[17] Paul, M., et al., Anthropogenic factors and the risk of highly pathogenic avian influenza H5N1: prospects from a spatial-based model. *Vet. Res.*, 2010. 41(3): p. 28.

[18] Souris, M., et al., Retrospective space-time analysis of H5N1 Avian Influenza emergence in Thailand. *Int. J. Health Geogr.*, 2010. 9: p. 3.

[19] Tiensin, T., et al., Ecologic risk factor investigation of clusters of avian influenza A (H5N1) virus infection in Thailand. *J. Infect Dis.,* 2009. 199(12): p. 1735-43.

[20] Gilbert, M., et al., Free-grazing ducks and highly pathogenic avian influenza, Thailand. *Emerg Infect Dis,* 2006. 12(2): p. 227-34.

[21] Gilbert, M., et al., Mapping H5N1 highly pathogenic avian influenza risk in Southeast Asia. *Proc. Natl. Acad. Sci. USA*, 2008. 105(12): p. 4769-74.

[22] Paul, M., et al., Risk factors for highly pathogenic avian influenza (HPAI) H5N1 infection in backyard chicken farms, Thailand. *Acta Trop*, 2011. 118(3): p. 209-16.

[23] Siengsanan, J., et al., Comparison of outbreaks of H5N1 highly pathogenic avian influenza in wild birds and poultry in Thailand. *J. Wildl Dis.*, 2009. 45(3): p. 740-7.

[24] Chantong, W. and J.B. Kaneene, Poultry raising systems and highly pathogenic avian influenza outbreaks in Thailand: the situation, associations, and impacts. *Southeast Asian J. Trop. Med. Public Health*, 2011. 42(3): p. 596-608.

[25] (DLD)., D.o.L.D., National Avian Influenza Surveillance System and Monitoring of Genetic Variations in Thailand. [Cited 2012 July 9]. Available from:http://www.dld.go.th/home/bird_flu/livestock_by_don/data/Control%20measures/National%20Avian%20Influenza%20.pdf.

[26] Bruschke, C. and B. Vallat, OIE standards and guidelines related to trade and poultry diseases. *Rev. Sci. Tech.*, 2008. 27(3): p. 627-32.

[27] Ratananakorn, L. and D. Wilson, Zoning and compartmentalisation as risk mitigation measures: an example from poultry production. *Rev. Sci. Tech.*, 2011. 30(1): p. 297-307.

[28] (OIE), W.O.f.A.H. Terrestrial Animal Health Code. Chapter 4.3.1. Zoning and compartmentalisation, 2011. [Cited 2012 July 10] Available at: http://www.oie.int/index.php?id=169andL=0andhtmfile=chapitre_1.4.3.htm.

[29] Thanawongnuwech, R., et al., Probable tiger-to-tiger transmission of avian influenza H5N1. *Emerg Infect Dis.*, 2005. 11(5): p. 699-701.

[30] Songserm, T., et al., Avian influenza H5N1 in naturally infected domestic cat. *Emerg Infect Dis.*, 2006. 12(4): p. 681-3.

[31] Choi, Y.K., et al., Studies of H5N1 influenza virus infection of pigs by using viruses isolated in Vietnam and Thailand in 2004. *J. Virol.*, 2005. 79(16): p. 10821-5.

[32] Liu, Y., et al., Susceptibility and transmissibility of pigeons to Asian lineage highly pathogenic avian influenza virus subtype H5N1. *Avian Pathol*, 2007. 36(6): p. 461-5.

[33] Jeong, O.M., et al., Experimental infection of chickens, ducks and quails with the highly pathogenic H5N1 avian influenza virus. *J. Vet. Sci.*, 2009. 10(1): p. 53-60.

[34] Brown, J.D., et al., Infectious and lethal doses of H5N1 highly pathogenic avian influenza virus for house sparrows (Passer domesticus) and rock pigeons (Columbia livia). *J. Vet. Diagn Invest*, 2009. 21(4): p. 437-45.

[35] Sun, H., et al., Pathogenicity in quails and mice of H5N1 highly pathogenic avian influenza viruses isolated from ducks. *Vet. Microbiol.*, 2011. 152(3-4): p. 258-65.

[36] Yamamoto, Y., et al., Limited susceptibility of pigeons experimentally inoculated with H5N1 highly pathogenic avian influenza viruses. *J. Vet. Med. Sci.*, 2012. 74(2): p. 205-8.

[37] Uchida, Y., et al., Molecular epidemiological analysis of highly pathogenic avian influenza H5N1 subtype isolated from poultry and wild bird in Thailand. *Virus Res.*, 2008. 138(1-2): p. 70-80.

[38] Chen, H., et al., Establishment of multiple sublineages of H5N1 influenza virus in Asia: implications for pandemic control. *Proc. Natl. Acad. Sci. USA*, 2006. 103(8): p. 2845-50.

[39] Toward a unified nomenclature system for highly pathogenic avian influenza virus (H5N1). *Emerg Infect Dis.*, 2008. 14(7): p. e1.

[40] Wang, J., et al., Identification of the progenitors of Indonesian and Vietnamese avian influenza A (H5N1) viruses from southern China. *J. Virol.*, 2008. 82(7): p. 3405-14.

[41] Wan, X.F., et al., Evolution of highly pathogenic H5N1 avian influenza viruses in Vietnam between 2001 and 2007. *PLoS One*, 2008. 3(10): p. e3462.

[42] Chaichoune, K., et al., Indigenous sources of 2007-2008 H5N1 avian influenza outbreaks in Thailand. *J. Gen. Virol.*, 2009. 90(Pt 1): p. 216-22.

[43] Smith, G.J., et al., Evolution and adaptation of H5N1 influenza virus in avian and human hosts in Indonesia and Vietnam. *Virology*, 2006. 350(2): p. 258-68.

[44] Cattoli, G., et al., Evidence for differing evolutionary dynamics of A/H5N1 viruses among countries applying or not applying avian influenza vaccination in poultry. *Vaccine,* 2011. 29(50): p. 9368-75.

[45] Amonsin, A., et al., Genetic characterization of 2008 reassortant influenza A virus (H5N1), Thailand. *Virol. J.*, 2010. 7: p. 233.

In: Avian Influenza
ISBN: 978-1-62417-415-5
Editors: K. M. Taylor and B. O'Connor

Chapter 4

How Quickly Did Bird Flu Go Off the Public Radar? Results of a Follow-up CATI Survey of Australian Adults

Sandra C. Jones*[*], *Don Iverson, Louise Waters, Max Sutherland, Julian Gold and Chris Puplick
Centre for Health Initiatives, University of Wollongong, Wollongong, New South Wales, Australia

Abstract

A survey of 200 Australian adults in May 2006 found reasonable levels of awareness, but low levels of concern, regarding bird flu. This paper reports on the changes in perceptions and attitudes that were identified in a follow-up survey conducted when bird flu was not the focus of widespread media coverage.

A computer assisted telephone survey was conducted in August and September 2006. A total of 5,565 eligible households were contacted and 805 interviews completed (response rate of 14.5%).

Bird flu fell from fourth to seventh most-frequently mentioned infectious disease. The majority of respondents were in favour of the

[*] Corresponding Author: Prof Sandra C Jones. Director, Centre for Health Initiatives, University of Wollongong. ITAMS Building, Innovation Campus, Wollongong NSW Australia. Ph: +61 2 4221 5106; Fax: +61 2 4221 3370; Email: sandraj@uow.edu.au.

government implementing quarantine procedures in the event of an outbreak, but less in favour of the government closing schools and offering people experimental vaccines or drugs. Respondents had low levels of awareness of preventive actions, but were generally willing to engage in these when they were identified.

We found that within four months of the initial high levels of concern bird flu was "off the radar" for the majority of the Australian population. One of the most important findings was that the general public appeared willing to engage in the appropriate preventive and protective behaviours, in the 'unlikely' event of a bird flu outbreak in Australia, but was lacking awareness of what these behaviours are.

Our results suggest that the Australian government will face a number of significant communication challenges in the event of an influenza pandemic. Not the least of these will be the need to communicate risk at the same time as educating people about appropriate preventive behaviours.

Avian influenza (commonly referred to as bird flu) was on the radar worldwide in 2005 following the identification of cases in humans, [1, 2] and health services and governments began planning for a potential avian influenza A (H5N1) pandemic. It was estimated, using clinical case rates from three previous influenza pandemics, that a bird flu pandemic would have likely case rates of between 24.7% and 34.2%, and death rates between 4.4 and 6.7 per 1000 people. [3] While H5N1 did not spread at the rate that was predicted by many, it was followed by a pandemic of H1N1 in 2009/10. [4-7]

In December 2008 the WHO released a revision of its pandemic influenza preparedness and response guidance document to assist countries in their planning and preparedness activities. [8] If a pandemic appears to be looming governments will have to act in a comprehensive and decisive manner to reduce the impact within their borders. [2,9] Any successful control efforts will require the cooperation of a country's residents – if coordinated actions are replaced by widespread public panic there is little hope of a pandemic being effectively managed.

Previous Studies of Knowledge and Perceptions of Emerging Infectious Diseases

A comprehensive search of academic databases conducted in early 2006 failed to locate any *published* population-based survey data concerning public knowledge and perceptions of avian influenza. However, there was data available online from two surveys conducted on a nationally representative sample of US residents by the Harvard School of Public Health, in January and September 2006. The January survey found that while 62% of the respondents were concerned about the possibility of a pandemic and 57% were concerned that it could spread to the US only 17% were very or somewhat worried about getting sick from it. Respondents were supportive of short-term quarantine for themselves if they had bird flu (96%) and indicated they would wash their hand more frequently (90%), reduce or avoid travel (75%), avoid public events or gatherings (71%), stay at home during the outbreak (68%) and wear a face mask (52%) if a human case occurred in the state in which they lived. [10] The September 2006 survey found that the public's estimation of the likelihood of a human case occurring in the US in the next 12 months had increased from 34% to 44%. The results again indicated strong support for recommended public health measures. [11]

Purpose of the Current Study

The authors conducted a population-based CATI survey of 200 Australian adults in May 2006; [12] at a time when there had been considerable media coverage of the potential for a bird flu pandemic. This paper reports on a follow-up study designed to (a) collect data from a larger sample; and (b) to determine whether there were any changes in the Australian public's knowledge, beliefs, attitudes, or willingness to engage in preventive behaviours since the initial survey was conducted in May 2006.

Methods

A computer assisted telephone survey (CATI) was conducted between 28th August and 14th September 2006. The sampling frame was the Desktop Marketing System (DTMS) which is a form of the electronic White Pages.

Of the 9,519 telephone numbers attempted, a total of 5,565 eligible households were contacted and 805 interviews were completed (response rate of 14.5%). Details of call attempts are provided in Table 1. The interview length averaged 12.36 minutes. Interviewing was conducted on weekdays between the hours of 4:30pm to 9:00pm and on weekends between 10:00am to 6:00pm.

Data was analysed using SPSS version 13.0. Inter-group comparisons were conducted for all questions, with the exception of those which elicited open-ended responses. For variables with two groups (e.g., gender and birth country), Mann-Whitney U (independent samples) tests were conducted; for variables with more than two groups (e.g. age category, income bracket), Kruskal-Wallis (non-parametric ANOVA) tests were conducted, with 10 and 7 degrees of freedom for age and income respectively.

A total of 805 respondents completed the survey; 55.0% (443) were female. Respondents were spread across all age groups, with 18.5% aged between 18 and 34; 17.5% aged 35 to 44; 23.3% aged 45 to 54; 18.9% aged 55 to 64; and 21.5% aged over 65. Just over three quarters (78.8%) were born in Australia. Approximately one third (32.7%) had completed less than five years of high school, 18.8% had completed five years, 12.1% a trade or other certificate, and 35.5% a diploma or degree. Approximately one quarter (23.4%) had an annual household income of less than $30,000, 30.4% between $30,000 and $70,000, 27.4% over $70,000, and 10.4% declined to provide household income information.

Table 1. Call attempts

Contact results	Total	NSW		VIC		QLD		SA		WA	
		Syd	Other NSW	Melb	Other VIC	Bris	Other QLD	Adel	Other SA	Per	Other WA
Interviews completed	805	120	121	120	121	60	60	60	40	62	41
Refused the interview	4760	1364	623	493	660	335	235	447	130	324	149
Language barrier	123	58	3	22	4	5	4	12	3	12	0
Unavailable in survey period	29	2	3	1	10	0	3	1	3	3	3
Quota full	253	62	34	8	57	7	7	21	2	33	22
Attempted but not contacted (< than 5 attempts)	1410	192	85	169	221	136	108	102	100	199	98
No answer after 5 attempts	82	1	16	53	4	0	6	1	0	1	0
Invalid Number (disconnected)	1822	441	185	216	186	121	118	151	64	212	128
Fax / Business	235	64	21	41	27	16	20	14	4	18	10
Total households	9519	2304	1091	1123	1290	680	561	809	346	864	451

Table 2. All disease mentions

	Survey 1			Survey 2		
	Male (%)	Female (%)	Total (%)	Male (%)	Female (%)	Total (%)
HIV/AIDS	45.0	39.0	41.9	45.0	37.7	41.0
Influenza (flu)	29.6	36.2	33.0	24.1	23.6	23.7
Measles/mumps/rubella	16.3	45.7	31.6	16.3	28.0	22.7
Hepatitis	18.4	18.2	18.3	19.9	23.2	21.7
Meningococcal disease	2.0	9.6	5.9	16.5	22.5	19.9
Chickenpox	5.0	17.2	11.3	5.9	17.9	12.4
Avian influenza (bird flu)	20.5	20.0	20.3	10.8	10.9	10.8
Cold	5.1	3.9	4.5	8.5	5.3	6.8
Tuberculosis	9.1	7.7	8.4	5.5	6.1	5.8
Malaria	2.0	-	1.0	3.3	1.6	2.4
Whooping cough	2.0	5.0	3.5	1.7	7.5	4.8
Sexually transmitted diseases	7.2	8.7	7.9	9.4	6.6	7.8
Staphylococcal infection	1.0	2.9	2.0	1.2	2.9	2.1
Meningitis	1.0	2.9	2.0	0.6	3.0	1.9
Polio	2.0	-	1.0	0.9	1.4	1.0
Cancer	1.0	1.0	1.0	3.4	0.7	1.7
Severe acute respiratory syndrome	1.0	2.0	1.5	2.0	1.4	1.6
Ross river virus	-	-	1.0	3.4	1.6	2.3
Pneumonia	3.0	1.0	2.0	1.5	1.4	1.4
Chlamydia	-	-	-	0.6	0.4	0.5
Diptheria	-	-	-	1.5	1.1	1.2
Typhoid	-	-	-	-	1.6	1.0
Smallpox	1.0	1.0	1.0	0.6	1.1	0.9
Glandular fever	-	-	-	0.6	1.3	0.9
Gastroenteritis	1.0	3.9	2.5	0.3	0.9	0.6
Other	11.2	19.1	14.9	18.6	20.6	20.0
Don't know/none	11.2	5.7	8.4	10.5	7.4	8.8

RESULTS

Respondents were first asked a general question about infectious diseases; "Living in Australia in 2006, what *infectious* diseases come to mind." respondents were able to nominate as many diseases as they wished; 8.8% were unable to name any infectious diseases (compared to 8.0% in survey one), 734 named one, 554 named more than one, and 310 named more than two. Data are first presented for all mentioned diseases for all respondents (Table 2) and then for the first mentioned (i.e. top of mind) diseases (Table 3).

The three most commonly mentioned diseases were HIV/AIDS (41.0%), influenza/flu (23.7%) and measles/mumps/rubella (22.7%); these were the same diseases, and in the same order, as in survey one.

Importantly, bird flu fell from fourth to seventh most-frequently mentioned disease, with only 10.8% of respondents (87) spontaneously mentioning bird flu, compared to 20.3% in survey one. In this survey, hepatitis (21.7%), meningococcal (19.9%) and chickenpox (12.4%) were all mentioned by more respondents than bird flu. In both surveys the primary difference between genders was that females were more likely to mention childhood diseases (such as measles/mumps/rubella and chickenpox) than were males.

Table 3. Top of mind disease mentions

	Survey 1 (%)	Survey 2 (%)
HIV/AIDS	22.2	23.4
Meningococcal disease (cerebrospinal meningitis)	4.9	10.6
Influenza (flu)	18.2	10.4
Hepatitis	6.9	8.0
Avian Influenza (bird flu)	14.3	5.2
Measles/mumps/rubella	8.4	5.0
Chicken pox	1.5	3.1
Cold	0.5	2.5
Tuberculosis	3.4	1.6
Whooping cough	0.5	1.4
Sexually transmitted diseases	3.4	1.2
Ross River fever	-	1.2
Cancer	1.0	1.0
Staphylococcal infection	1.5	0.9
Malaria	0.5	0.9
Meningitis	-	0.7
SARS (Severe Acute Respiratory Syndrome)	-	0.6
Diptheria	-	0.4
Polio	-	0.2
Typhoid	-	0.2
Fever	-	0.2
Other	4.5	12.3
Don't know/none	8.4	8.8
Total	100.0	100.0

For top-of-mind (first) responses, HIV/AIDS was the most common in both surveys. However, whereas flu in general and bird flu specifically were the next highest top of mind responses in survey one (18.2% and 14.3% respectively), these were significantly lower in survey to (10.4% and 5.2% respectively). In survey two, meningococcal disease was the second most common response (10.6%), perhaps reflecting recent media coverage of high profile meningococcal cases, and bird flu had dropped from third to fifth place behind hepatitis (8.0%).

Table 4. Infectious diseases of most concern

	Male	Female	Total	Male	Female	Total
Meningococcal disease	2.0	6.7	4.4	10.7	18.0	14.8
HIV/AIDS	18.4	17.1	17.7	14.2	12.6	13.4
Influenza (flu)	13.3	16.2	14.8	12.9	10.1	11.4
Hepatitis	9.2	5.7	7.4	6.8	8.8	7.9
Avian influenza (bird flu)	12.2	9.5	10.8	7.7	3.8	5.6
Measles/mumps/rubella	1.0	5.7	3.4	2.5	2.0	2.2
Cold	1.0	1.9	1.5	2.7	1.3	1.9
Tuberculosis	2.0	1.0	1.5	1.9	1.3	1.6
Chickenpox	-	1.9	1.0	0.5	2.2	1.5
Whooping cough	-	-	-	0.3	2.0	1.2
Ross river fever	-	-	-	1.4	1.1	1.2
Cancer	-	-	-	2.2	0.4	1.2
Meningitis	1.0	1.0	1.0	0.3	1.6	1.0
Staphylococcal infection	1.0	2.9	2.0	0.3	1.3	0.9
Gastroenteritis	1.0	1.9	1.5	-	-	-
Sexually transmitted diseases	2.0	1.0	1.5	1.1	0.7	0.9
Pneumonia	-	-	-	0.8	0.2	0.5
Malaria	-	-	-	0.5	0.2	0.4
Viral infections	-	-	-	-	0.4	0.2
Typhoid	-	-	-	-	0.4	0.2
Polio	-	-	-	-	0.4	0.2
Other	6.1	4.9	5.5	6.9	9.0	7.8
Don't know/none	29.6	22.9	26.1	26.3	22.2	24.2
Total			100.0	100.0	100.0	100.0

Respondents were then asked which of these are of *greatest* concern to them (Table 4). The list of diseases of greatest concern was similar to the list of diseases that come to mind. Thus, the disease of greatest concern was meningococcal disease (14.8%), compared to only 4.4% in survey one. Among the other most concerning diseases were HIV/AIDS (13.4% in survey two and 17.7% in survey one) and influenza/flu (11.4% in survey two and 14.8% in survey one). The drop in spontaneous mentions of bird flu was reflected in a drop in the proportion of respondents identifying this is the disease of most concern (from 10.8% to 5.6% in survey two).

Perceived Risk of, and Concern about, Bird Flu

Respondents were then read the following sentence: "One infectious disease that has been in the media lately is bird flu. Thinking now about the *bird flu*, as far as you know, has bird flu ever been spread from human to human?" Just over one quarter (27.3%) of respondents answered yes to this question, with 55.2% answering no, and 17.5% that they didn't know.

All respondents were then asked how likely they thought it was that bird flu would spread from human to human in Australia within the next 12 months. As shown in Table 5, there was a far lower level of agreement that this would be the case in Australia, with only less than quarter of respondents believing that it is either very likely (4.7%) or somewhat likely (17.6%) which reflects a slight reduction between the two surveys (from 26.1% in survey one to 22.3% in survey two). Again, female respondents were more likely than males to believe this would occur ($z = -3.64$, $p = .000$) and, again, the same pattern was observed in survey one ($Z = -1.75$, $p = .08$).

Table 5. Perceived likelihood that bird flu will spread from human to human in Australia

	Survey 1 (%)	Survey 2 (%)
Very likely	3.9	4.7
Somewhat likely	22.2	17.6
Somewhat unlikely	27.6	29.6
Very unlikely	40.4	42.2
(Not sure)	5.9	5.8
Total	100.0	100.0

Respondents were next asked how concerned they were that they or someone in their immediate family might catch bird flu. As shown in Table 6, less than one quarter of respondents reported that they were very concerned (7.2%) or somewhat concerned (14.0%); this reflects a slight reduction from survey one (from 23.6% somewhat or very concerned in survey one to 21.2% in survey two). The biggest change between the two surveys was a sizeable increase in the proportion reporting that they are not at all concerned that they or someone in their family might catch bird flu (from 36.9% in survey one to 45.7% in survey two).

Unlike survey one, there was a significant gender difference, with female respondents more likely to report being concerned (Z = -2.80, p = .005). Older respondents were more likely to report being concerned (χ^2 = 26.50, p = .003), although this trend was only apparent up until the age of 60 (with the 60-64 and 65+ age groups much less concerned); survey one also found that younger respondents tended to be slightly less concerned than older respondents about someone in their family catching bird flu (χ^2 = 17.8, p = .06). There was also an association between level of concern and household income, such that as those on higher incomes reported being *less concerned* about themselves or a family member catching bird flu (χ^2 = 16.58, p = .02).

Table 6. Concern that respondent or someone in their family might catch bird flu

	Survey 1 (%)	Survey 2 (%)
Very concerned	10.8	7.2
Somewhat concerned	12.8	14.0
Not too concerned	39.4	32.5
Not at all concerned	36.9	45.7
Not sure (NOT READ OUT)		.5
Total	100.0	100.0

Knowledge and Attitudes Related to Bird Flu

When asked how likely they believe it was that they would die from bird flu if they were to catch it, it was evident that the majority perceived this disease to be fatal. As shown in Table 7, over two thirds of respondents believed that, were they to catch bird flu, they would be either very likely (33.2 %) or somewhat likely (35.3 %) to die from it. Again, these figures are extremely consistent with those from survey one (32.0% and 36.9% respectively). Female respondents reported thinking it is more likely that someone will die from bird flu than male respondents (Z = -2.66, p = .008), a difference which was not evident in survey one.

Table 7. Perceived likelihood of dying from bird flu if contracted

	Survey 1 (%)	Survey 2 (%)
Very likely	32.0	33.2
Somewhat likely	36.9	35.3
Somewhat unlikely	9.4	15.7
Very unlikely	11.8	7.0
Not sure (NOT READ OUT)	9.9	8.9
Total	100.0	100.0

Current and Potential Engagement in Protective Actions

Respondents were first asked about things the government might do to control an outbreak of bird flu if it were to spread among humans. They were read a list of items and asked whether they would favour or oppose the government taking each of the potential actions. For two of the actions included the wording was slightly altered in survey two.

As shown in Table 8, the majority of respondents were in favour of the government quarantining those who had been exposed to bird flu (95.8% in favour and 3.2% opposed), closing the borders to visitors from countries where people have bird flu (83.2% in favour and 14.2% opposed), and requiring people to work from home when possible (83.7% in favour and 13.3% opposed); with these figures relatively unchanged from survey one. However, they were less in favour of the government closing schools (74.9% in favour and 21.5% opposed) and offering people experimental vaccines or drugs (69.9% in favour and 23.4% opposed); although, in contrast to the previous actions, the proportion in favour had increased considerably since survey one (from 65.5% to 74.9% in favour of closing schools, and from 54.2% to 69.9% in favour of experimental vaccines or drugs).

Table 8. Support for hypothetical government actions in the event of an outbreak

	Survey1		Survey 2	
	Favour (%)	Oppose (%)	Favour (%)	Oppose (%)
Require (encourage) people to work from home when possible	74.9	21.2	83.7	13.3
Quarantine those who have been exposed to bird flu	96.1	2.5	95.8	3.2
Close the borders to visitors from countries where people have bird flu (with outbreaks)	81.8	13.8	83.2	14.2
Close schools	65.5	27.1	74.9	21.5
Offer people experimental vaccines or drugs	54.2	35.5	69.9	23.4

There were significant differences between male and female respondents on three of the five items, and in all three cases females were more in favour of the listed actions: require people to work from home if they are able ($Z = -3.24$, $p = .001$); quarantine those who have been exposed to bird flu ($Z = -2.13$, $p = .03$); and close borders to visitors from countries where people have bird flu ($Z = -2.14$, $p = .03$).

Respondents were then asked what actions they thought would be *their* highest priority to protect themselves and their families in the event of an outbreak of bird flu in Australia. The most commonly mentioned actions (Table 9) were to enquire about or have a vaccine (24.4%), avoid people or places who might be infected (22.7%), and to isolate or quarantine themselves (21.9%). A small proportion of respondents spontaneously mentioned two of the actions which are actually most likely to reduce the spread of bird flu; washing hands more frequently (3.5%, if we optimistically assume that is what people meant when they referred to personal hygiene) and wearing face masks (5.5%). However, none of the respondents mentioned using disposable tissues rather than handkerchiefs.

Respondents were then asked which actions they would be willing to take in the event that the government warned there was an increased risk of bird flu among humans and specifically recommended that they took those actions. Respondents were asked to indicate their willingness by a yes or no response. Given this scenario, the actions which respondents stated they would be most willing to engage in were to increase hand washing (88.2%), clean items they share with other people (87.7%), ask their doctor for prescriptions for a flu vaccine or antiviral drugs (85.0%), and change their holiday travel plans

(83.9%). Further, 73.3 % said they would be prepared to change from use of handkerchiefs to use of disposable tissues which, when combined with the 13.8% who stated that they already used disposable tissues exclusively, shows that the majority of the population (87.1%) would be prepared to engage in this behaviour (see Table 10). However, there were several actions which a large proportion of the respondents stated they would not be prepared to take, including avoiding physical contact with people such as shaking hands (28.7%), wearing face masks in public (25.8%), working from home (19.0%), keeping their children home from school (18.9%), and changing their business travel plans (18.3%).

Table 9. Spontaneously mentioned high priority actions

	Frequency	Percent
Enquire/have vaccine	197	24.4
Avoid crowds/places/people who might be infected	183	22.7
Isolation/quarantine myself/everyone	176	21.9
Go to see a doctor/seek medical advice	54	6.7
Find more information/educate myself about it	54	6.7
Wearing a mask	44	5.5
Stop/consume less chicken	34	4.2
Avoid contact with all birds	29	3.6
Take care of personal hygiene/cleanliness	28	3.5
Follow the government/federal/health department's instructions	24	3.0
Look after your health/have a balanced diet	16	2.0
Avoid contact with chickens	12	1.5
Prevent getting infected/spreading	11	1.4
Not planning/going overseas	11	1.4
Nothing/carry on with my normal life	10	1.2
Move/run away from contaminated areas	10	1.2
Exterminate all chickens	9	1.1
Exterminate all birds	7	0.9
Stock up food/drink	6	0.7
Other	24	3.0
Don't know/not sure	105	13
Total	805	100.0

Table 10. Willingness to take preventive actions if advised by the government

	Yes (%)	No (%)	Not sure (%)	Total (%)
Increase hand washing	88.2	10.9	0.9	100.0
Clean items you share with other people (e.g. telephones)	87.7	10.9	1.4	100.0
Ask your doctor for prescriptions for a flu vaccine, Tamiflu, Relenza, or other antiviral drugs	85.0	12.0	3.0	100.0
Change holiday travel plans	83.9	13.8	2.4	100.0
Work from home	77.5	19.0	3.5	100.0
Change business travel plans	77.0	18.3	4.7	100.0
Keep your children home from school	74.0	18.9	7.1	100.0
Change from use of handkerchiefs to use of disposable tissues	73.3	12.4	0.5	86.3*
Wear face masks in public	69.9	25.8	4.2	100.0
Avoid physical contact with people (e.g., shaking hands)	67.2	28.7	4.1	100.0

* 13.8% (111) stated that they already use paper tissues only.

Of the five items worded identically in the two surveys, we noted an increase in the proportion of respondents stating that they would be willing to engage in all five: increase hand washing (from 83.3% in survey one to 88.2% in survey two), clean items they share with other people (from 71.4% to 87.7%), ask their doctor for prescriptions for a flu vaccine or antiviral drugs (from 60.1% to 85.0%), avoid physical contact with people such as shaking hands (from 41.9% to 67.2%), and (continue or) change to use of disposable tissues (from 79.3% to 86.3%). For the two items with modified wording in both cases the wording was strengthened, making any estimate of change in attitudes conservative: willingness to wear face masks in survey two (69.9%) was higher than the willingness simply to purchase these in survey one (55.7%); and willingness to keep children home from school in survey two (74.0%) was higher than to "make plans" to do so in survey one (57.6%).

There were significant differences between male and female respondents on eight of the ten items, and in all eight cases females reported greater willingness to engage in the recommended actions: increase hand washing ($Z = 2.34$, $p = .02$); clean items shared with other people ($Z = 2.32$, $p = .02$);

change holiday travel plans (Z = 2.44, p = .02); change business travel plans (Z = 3.63, p = .000); keep children home from school (Z = 2.47, p = .01); change from use of handkerchiefs to use of disposable tissues (Z = 3.14, p = .002); wear face masks in public (Z = 2.23, p = .03); and avoid physical contact with people (Z = 4.19, p = .000).

Respondents were then asked where they would go for diagnosis and/or treatment in the event that they thought that they or a member of their family had been infected with bird flu (this was an unprompted response, recorded verbatim and post-coded, and respondents could give more than one option). As shown in Table 11, the most common response was their local GP or family doctor (58.1%), followed by the hospital emergency room (34.2%).

Table 11. Anticipated sources of diagnosis and/or treatment

	Frequency	Percent
Your local GP/family doctor	468	58.0
Hospital emergency	275	34.0
Hospital	27	3.4
Infectious disease hospital/ clinic	26	3.2
Specialist	14	1.7
Medical centre/health clinic	10	1.2
Department of health/ government	10	1.2
Ring the infectious disease hotline	4	0.5
Ring 000	4	0.5
Internet	2	0.2
Other	40	5.0
Don't know	3	0.4

DISCUSSION

Awareness of Bird Flu

The first, and perhaps most important, finding from this second CATI survey was that bird flu was "off the radar" for the majority of the Australian population. Looking at all mentions, bird flu fell from the fourth to the seventh most-frequently mentioned disease (from 20.3% in May to 10.8% of respondents in September), meaning that for 90% of the population surveyed bird flu was not even considered as an infectious disease worthy of mention by

September 2006. Further, top of mind mentions fell dramatically for both bird flu specifically and flu in general. This finding was consistent with that of Watkins and colleagues [13] who conducted three focus groups with 23 owners/senior managers of small and medium businesses in Perth, Australia; none of the 23 participants spontaneously identified bird flu as being an important health issue for their businesses.

HIV/AIDS was, by most measures, the disease which received both the highest awareness and the highest level of concern across both surveys. The findings in relation to meningococcal disease were surprising, and add considerable support to the often-stated view that the media serves an agenda setting function in relation to health and medical issues. All mentions of meningococcal disease increased from 5.9% in May to 19.9% in September; top of mind mentions increased from 4.9% to 10.6%; and mentions of meningococcal disease as the disease of most concern increased from 4.4% to 14.8% (surpassing even HIV/AIDS). We conducted a retrospective search of Australian and New Zealand newsprint coverage (using the Factiva database) for the periods 01 April to 31 May and 01 August to 30 September 2006, and found that in the former period there were 68 articles relating to meningococcal disease and in the latter period 238 (that is, almost four times as many). It is reasonable to assume that the increase in awareness and concern for meningococcal disease was a result of this high level of media coverage of the condition.

Bird Flu Knowledge and Attitudes

We found an increase in the proportion of respondents believing that it is very or somewhat likely that bird flu will spread from human to human, but a *decrease* in the proportion who believed this would occur in Australia. Perhaps reflecting this sense of confidence that bird flu would not travel to Australia, less than one quarter reported feeling concerned that someone in their family would contract bird flu.

Bird Flu Prevention and Precautions

One of the most important findings from this research was that the general public appeared willing to engage in the appropriate preventive and protective behaviours, but was lacking awareness of what these behaviours are. That is, respondents' spontaneous mentions of high priority actions to protect themselves and their families were vaccination (although there was at that point no vaccine available for bird flu) and avoiding infected others or quarantining themselves. As reported above, only a very small proportion of respondents spontaneously mentioned hand washing or wearing face masks, and none mentioned use of disposable tissues. However, when asked about their willingness to engage in these behaviours were they advised to do so, almost 90% responded that they would be willing to engage in more frequent hand washing and change to the exclusive use of disposable tissues, and almost 70% that they would be willing to wear face masks. Further, for those protective actions also included in the previous survey, this survey showed small increases in the proportion stating willingness to engage in all five behaviours (increase hand washing, clean items shared with other people, ask doctor for prescriptions for a flu vaccine or antiviral drugs, avoid physical contact with people such as shaking hands, and (continue or) change to use of disposable tissues). The Perth study noted that while the business owners /managers were concerned about the impact of a pandemic on their businesses they had not engaged in preparedness planning nor were they planning to, but they wanted information regarding what they could do in the event of a pandemic. [13]

However, there were several actions which more than one in five of the respondents stated they would not be prepared to take, including avoiding physical contact with people such as shaking hands, wearing face masks in public, working from home, keeping their children home from school, and changing their business travel plans. As these responses were in relation to a hypothetical outbreak (which respondents perceived as unlikely), it is possible that the reported willingness underestimates the level of agreement that would exist in the event that this actually occurred; a recent survey of households in North Carolina following a closure of schools during an Influenza B outbreak found that 91% of respondents were in favour of the closure. [14] However, in this Australian sample, the behaviours that people stated they would be unwilling to engage in appeared to fall into two categories; actions which people may not believe they are personally able to control primarily due to work commitments (working from home, changing business travel plans, and keeping children home from school), and actions with social implications (wearing face masks in public and avoiding physical contact).

Conclusion/Implications

Our results suggest that, as was the case with the SARS outbreaks in Canada and Hong Kong, the Australian government will face a number of significant communication challenges in the event of a pandemic influenza outbreak. At the height of government and health agency concern about potential pandemic avian influenza the Australian public had a low level of awareness of, and concern about, bird flu; while they perceived the disease to be fatal they did not perceive it as one which posed risks to people living in Australia. If there is an outbreak of pandemic influenza that reaches Australia, the government will be faced with needing to communicate to a scared public the nature and importance of the appropriate preventive health measures while at the same time seeking not to encourage public panic and inappropriate behavioural responses. We recommend that there should be at least two components of any communication strategy – one that prepares the public in the event of an influenza outbreak overseas or an increased risk of transmission in Australia, and one that directs persons to take specific actions during the actual outbreak. On this latter point it is encouraging to note that when the public actually encounters an infectious disease outbreak they are much more likely comply with recommended control measures. [15] However, it is equally important that this awareness-raising does not happen too far in advance of cases occurring in Australia as our results suggest that communicating risk in advance of its emergence, at least via the mass media, results in the public discounting the reality of the risk.

Acknowledgments

This research was funded by the National Health and Medical Research Council under the Council's Urgent Research Scheme.

References

[1] Wulandari F, Lyn TE. *Indonesia struggles to track H5N1 source, two more die,* 2006 [cited 2007 June 01] Available from www.medscape.com/viewarticle/532937.

[2] Butler D. Pandemic 'dry run' is cause for concern. *Nature.* 2006; 441(7094):554-555. DOI:10.1038/441554a.

[3] Brundage JF. Cases and deaths during influenza pandemics in the United States. *Am J Prev Med.* 2006; 31(3):252-256. DOI: 10.1016/j.amepre.2006.04.005.

[4] Viboud, C. & Simonsen, L. Global mortality of 2009 pandemic influenza A H1N1. *The Lancet Infectious Diseases,* 2012. 12(9): 651-653.

[5] Valenciano M, Kissling E, Cohen J-M, Oroszi B, Barret A-S, et al. Estimates of Pandemic Influenza Vaccine Effectiveness in Europe, 2009–2010: Results of Influenza Monitoring Vaccine Effectiveness in Europe (I-MOVE) Multicentre Case-Control Study. *PLoS Med* 8(1): e1000388.doi:10.1371/journal.pmed.1000388.

[6] Brandt C, Rabenau HF, Bornmann S, Gottschalk R, Wicker S. The impact of the 2009 influenza A(H1N1) pandemic on attitudes of healthcare workers toward seasonal influenza vaccination 2010/11. *Euro Surveill.* 2011;16(17):pii=19854. Available online: http://www.eurosurveillance.org/ViewArticle.aspx?ArticleId=19854

[7] Andradottir S, Chiu W, Goldsman D, Lee ML, Tsui K-L, Sander B, Fisman DN & Nizam A. Reactive strategies for containing developing outbreaks of pandemic influenza. BMC Public Health 2011, 11(Suppl 1):S1 doi:10.1186/1471-2458-11-S1-S1.

[8] World Health Organization. Pandemic influenza preparedness and response. 2009 [cited 2012 Sept 05] Available from http://whqlibdoc.who.int/publications/2009/9789241547680_eng.pdf.

[9] Mounier-Jack S, Coker RJ. How prepared is Europe for pandemic influenza? Analysis of national plans. *Lancet North Am Ed.* 2006; 367(9520):1405-1411. DOI:10.1016/S0140-6736(06)68511-5.

[10] Blendon RJ, Benson JM, Fleischfresser C, Weldon KJ, Herrmann MJ. Avian flu survey: January 17-25, 2006 [cited 2012 August 25] Available from http://www.hsph.harvard.edu/disasters/articles/Loree-Blendon.pdf.

[11] Blendon RJ, Benson JM, Weldon KJ, Herrmann MJ. Pandemic influenza survey: September 28-October 5, 2006 [cited 2012 August 25] Available from http://www.hsph.harvard.edu/news/press-releases/2006-releases/press10262006.html.

[12] Jones SC, Iverson D. What Australians know and believe about bird flu: results of a population telephone survey, *Health Prom Prac.* 2008; 9(4 Supplement): 73S-82S.

[13] Watkins RE, Cooke FC, Donovan RJ, MacIntyre R, Itzwerth R, Plant AJ. Tackle the problem when it gets here: pandemic preparedness among small and medium businesses. *Qual Health Res.* 2008; 18:902-912. DOI: 10.1177/1049732308318032.

[14] Johnson AJ, Moore ZS, Edelson PJ, Kinnane L, Davies M, Shay DK, Balish A, McCarron M, Blanton L, Finelle L, Averhoff F, Bresee J, Engel J, Fiore A. Household Responses to School Closure Resulting from Outbreak of Influenza B, North Carolina. *Emerg Infect Dis.* 2008; 14(7):1024-1030. DOI: 10.3201/eid1407.080096.

[15] Blendon RJ, Benson JM, DesRoches CM, Raleigh E, Taylor-Clark K. The public's response to severe acute respiratory syndrome in Toronto and the United States. *Clin Infect Dis.* 2004; 38: 925-31.

INDEX

F

G

H

I

J

K

L

M

N

O

P

T

U

V

W